# Hilary Ann

## A Broken Heart

### Daniel J. Dyman, Ed.D.

Order this book online at www.trafford.com/07-1411
or email orders@trafford.com

Most Trafford titles are also available at major online book retailers.

© Copyright 2007 Daniel J. Dyman Ed.D
27916 Crestview Drive, Elkhart, IN 46517
All rights reserved. No part of this publication may be reproduced, stored in a retrieval system, or transmitted, in any form or by any means, electronic, mechanical, photocopying, recording, or otherwise, without the written prior permission of the author.

Note for Librarians: A cataloguing record for this book is available from Library and Archives Canada at www.collectionscanada.ca/amicus/index-e.html

Printed in Victoria, BC, Canada.

ISBN: 978-1-4251-3612-3

We at Trafford believe that it is the responsibility of us all, as both individuals and corporations, to make choices that are environmentally and socially sound. You, in turn, are supporting this responsible conduct each time you purchase a Trafford book, or make use of our publishing services. To find out how you are helping, please visit www.trafford.com/responsiblepublishing.html

Our mission is to efficiently provide the world's finest, most comprehensive book publishing service, enabling every author to experience success. To find out how to publish your book, your way, and have it available worldwide, visit us online at www.trafford.com/10510

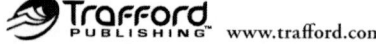 www.trafford.com

**North America & international**
toll-free: 1 888 232 4444 (USA & Canada)
phone: 250 383 6864 ♦ fax: 250 383 6804 ♦ email: info@trafford.com

**The United Kingdom & Europe**
phone: +44 (0)1865 722 113 ♦ local rate: 0845 230 9601
facsimile: +44 (0)1865 722 868 ♦ email: info.uk@trafford.com

10 9 8 7 6 5 4 3

to
My Father
for all of the blessings
I have received through him

and as well to all of those special people who recognized
Hilary Ann as a citizen of this world as she was with
special needs and deserving of care.

Hilary Ann gave us the opportunity to be at our very best,
to be most noble measuring up to whatever was required.

# DISCLAIMER

*This work,* Hilary Ann – A Broken Heart, *is non-fiction. Any association or any resemblance to historical events; names or people living or dead; places and locations; and incidents or events portrayed in this story is coincidental.*

# 1

Perhaps for us the storm of January 6, 1976, was an omen of the tragedy that was about to unfold.

It was exactly 4:30 p.m. I had just wrapped up work for my Biology 101 laboratory class. My office telephone was ringing. As I answered the call, Charlene broke into my greeting, "Dan, Dr. Earl agreed to see me at the hospital. Get home as soon as you can. Please!"

I responded, "I'll see you as quickly as I can get there."

Without a moment of hesitation, I hung up the telephone, grabbed my coat, and pulled the office door shut allowing it to slam behind me. As I hurriedly made my way through the hallway, I began to run at the building exit and across the parking lot to my heavy-duty pick-up truck.

This had been the fifth time Charlene called me. She had not been feeling well throughout the day experiencing cramps and general discomfort. The doctor had been putting her off. That would have been easy for him to do because Charlene had been conditioned to abide by whatever she was "supposed" to do.

However, with an unwavering mindset to get home driving as fast as conditions would permit, I felt grateful that Charlene had persisted.

She did call the doctor one more time as I had urged saying to her, "Insist that you need a check up. Cry if you have to. That's reasonable and the doctor ought to understand. He has to. If nothing is wrong, we at least would have some assurance and we would just come home."

Today, the drive would take at least twenty-five minutes if not longer through difficult snow covered country roads.

Daniel J. Dyman, Ed.D.

I wasted no time in clearing snow from the windows. A quick brush was enough for me to get going. In a second, I started the engine and was on my way.

We lived in a snow-belt region and it had been snowing throughout the day on top of several inches that already had accumulated. Throughout the day, the westerly wind had been brisk causing some serious drifting. Our house was set back from the road giving us a wonderful front yard but on a day like today our driveway, about 250 feet long, might be impassable. At its entrance, I probably should have had a winter sign, "Enter At Your Own Risk."

As I arrived, it was terrible. However, without a second thought, I turned the truck into the driveway. That might have been a poor choice but I was determined to make it to the back of our house. The snow was almost to the middle of the wheels but now in low gear, I managed.

Charlene had been waiting at the back door. Upon seeing me, she began waving and pointing toward the inside of the house, she shouted just barely over the roar of the truck, "My mother is here."

I responded with a "thumbs up" gesture coupled with a nod and a bless-her-heart smile.

Her mother had arrived just a few minutes earlier. She had walked from down the road to take care of the girls, Shellie, four months beyond six years old, and Therese, not quite sixteen months.

Throughout the day Charlene had been desperately trying to be in touch with her mother who earlier had been aimlessly shopping and then visiting with a neighbor not reachable by telephone. Thankfully, in time, she had just made it home. She was our only babysitter. At the moment we felt fortunate that her mother would be with the girls.

## Hilary Ann – A Broken Heart

Now, having to take the children with us was not a concern. The truck had only a single bench seat, not enough room to safely sit the girls between us though they were small in stature. We would have had to take our less snow worthy car parked in the garage.

At the moment all was going well. I was both thankful and relieved.

As I was spinning the wheels to turn around, Charlene began making her way toward the truck through a patch of drifted snow that was almost to her knees. Before the truck could come to a complete stop, with concern upon her face, she was tugging to open the passenger door.

Immediately upon stepping up into the truck, Charlene began to complain. "Dr. Earl doesn't believe the baby is coming. But, thank God, he agreed to check me at the hospital. He thinks I'm overreacting because the baby isn't due until the first week of March. Just flat out he said to me, 'You're not having your baby today!'"

I listened as we began the long drive to County Hospital.

Charlene continued, "As you know, I called him this morning telling him that something was wrong. He wouldn't listen. He said, 'The baby isn't due for several weeks.' He told me to keep my feet elevated. I did. But, this afternoon when the pains continued and got more frequent, I called him as you insisted. You were right. This isn't the first baby I have had."

Charlene began sobbing, "Something isn't right. I know it. And, of all things, I forgot my overnight bag. I left it in the kitchen. If I have the baby, you'll have to go back to get it for me."

My effort was concentrated on driving but in my silence, I did agree with Charlene. Her beliefs about having the baby could not be questioned. A moment later, I assured her that if needed, getting her overnight bag would not be a problem.

When finally we arrived at the hospital emergency room, some forty-five minutes after starting out from our house, the nurse from the obstetric unit checked Charlene and confirmed that she was in labor.

With a certain smile the nurse added, "Likely, it'll be a few hours."

Without hesitation, I said, "I'll be back as soon as I can."

I gave Charlene a little hug and without any more to-do started for the things she had left behind. I thought, "If you don't leave immediately, if you were to wait even for a short while, likely you will not make it home let alone return to the hospital."

During the few minutes that I had been in the hospital, neither the wind nor the snow had let up. The road conditions would become even more treacherous because the dreary atmosphere of the day was beginning to give way to nightfall. Driving would become steadily more difficult. In the darkness of country roads, headlights would be of little help if any at all. As anticipated, even when using the low beams, the light reflected by the snowflakes was blinding.

Through wooded areas, the bigger trees broke the wind but as I approached the last long north and south stretch of road bounded on either side by smaller orchard trees, the blowing snow became nearly impossible. Visibility was down to zero. I could not see beyond the front end of the truck. Suddenly, panic stricken, my heart began to race. I had hit a drift and ended up two rows deep in the midst of an orchard of now shadowy and ghostly appearing apple trees, maybe fifty feet off the road. In a single breath I responded, shifting into a lower gear. Intensity increased. I felt lucky as I kept the truck going driving through the rows of trees. As the truck fishtailed time and again, I cut the wheels. Again, I was determined.

My mental voice said, "Don't let up. Be watchful. You can't lose control. You can't hit one of those trees."

I realized that if the truck were to lose momentum, even just a little, I would not make it back to the hospital. I would need a tow to get out, at best maybe in a day or two.

I continued on looking for any opening to get back on the road. As each moment passed dodging trees, I tried to inch closer and closer to the roadway.

Unexpectedly, I felt the truck rise up out of the snow. I had made it to an elevation, probably an access drive. The snow seemed not as deep. Immediately, I reacted turning the wheels sharply toward the road. In a heartbeat, I swerved again. I was on the roadway going in the right direction.

In a state of absolute elation, I shouted, "Yes! Thank God for guardian angels. You made it."

My mental voice added, "Only a single right turn at the next intersection and two miles to go. But you will have to get back. With each passing minute, the roads are only getting worse."

At the moment, all that really mattered was that Charlene was at the hospital. If I were unable to make it back, the people there could provide for her every need.

I stopped at the entrance to the driveway. This time I decided not to gamble as before. The snow appeared to be too deep. The wheel tracks from less than two hours earlier had been drifted over. Rather than take a chance on getting stuck, I left the truck in the road with bright lights on and flashers blinking. I ran to the house.

Out of breath, I gave the girls a hug and reassured Charlene's mom that everything was okay. I grabbed Charlene's bag and bounded through the snow, trying to land in the footstep depressions I had just made going the opposite direction. In seconds it seemed I was in the truck and going again.

Rather than turn the truck around in the roadway, the better option was to drive straight on to a crossroad a little out of the way and then cut back as I could to the main road I had just used to and from the hospital. Again, I became tense. I was not sure that I would be able to make it back. In only a few moments, the wind seemed to have picked up. The snow appeared to be blowing more than before. When I got back to the main road, my tire tracks from moments ago were almost snow covered. Obviously, no other vehicles had been on the road. Because I knew the way, I was able to stay on course by measuring my distance from the mailboxes and trees that lined the road. I drove the truck to go as fast as the conditions would allow.

My only concern was for Charlene and the baby. Hopefully, they would be okay.

Thoughts flooded my mind, "Obviously, the doctor had miscalculated. Could he be that far off? No matter what, the girls at home will be fine. Watch the road. Keep the truck going smoothly. You have to get to the hospital, to be on time to for the delivery."

When my mind was quiet, I prayed that everything would continue to go well.

After what seemed to be an eternity, I could see the lights from County Hospital. Their glow was reassuring. The voice in my mind said, "Thank God." I knew that I would make it even if I would have to walk the rest of the way. I felt a sense of accomplishment, maybe of victory. The return trip took nearly an hour.

As I arrived at the nurse's station, the ward clerk looked up, smiled, and said, "Your wife is doing fine. You'll find her in room 114."

A nearby nurse added, "Things have slowed down a bit but it shouldn't be too much longer."

Hearing that, I felt some relief. I returned a polite smile. My heart was pounding. Still out of breath I said, "Thank you."

It was 7:55 p.m. when I walked into Charlene's labor room. As I entered, I heard her say to me with some unsettledness in her voice, "All is well so far."

I answered, "I'm glad."

I could see that Charlene was uncomfortable.

With an accommodating smile and a detectable groan and gasp in her voice, she continued, "How are you doing?"

As I pulled up a chair next to her bed, I replied, "I made it. That's all that matters. I'm just grateful to be here with you."

The labor had subsided. Every fifteen minutes, for the next few hours, the nurse returned to check Charlene. Each time just before leaving she would gesture waving with her right hand index finger pointing upward, smile, and cheerfully say, "We're coming along."

Just a little past 10:30 p:m. the labor intensified. "Get ready," was the nurse's comment.

She began preparing Charlene for the delivery. I was given a gown, cap, mask, and booties. I instantly arose. I dressed as quickly as I could and followed the nurse who wheeled Charlene into the delivery room.

## Daniel J. Dyman, Ed.D.

Dr. Earl, the Obstetrics and Gynecology physician, was on the way. His residence was a few blocks away from the hospital, only minutes in walking distance.

When the doctor arrived, the delivery procedures began. I stood off to the side watching. The time past unnoticed. At 11:14 p.m. Hilary Ann was born, five pounds, seven and one half ounces. Her name had been chosen the day after Charlene learned that she was pregnant.

But, rather than the excitement I had witnessed with the other children, Dr. Earl was in a frenzy. He was thumping Hilary on her chest, jostling her. She was not crying.

He placed Hilary on a small isolette and hurriedly began to examine her, listening for heart sounds. I could see that she was breathing and that she was taking on a pink coloration. However, Dr. Earl's every action showed concern. Oxygen was brought in followed by an incubator.

Charlene was straining to see what was going on. As tears began to fill her eyes, she called out, "The baby isn't crying. What's wrong? Is the baby okay? Is the baby okay? Please tell me."

Neither Dr. Earl nor either of the nurses responded. They continued in their preoccupation.

Our concern continued but as moments passed it began to give way to a more worrisome anticipation. We watched and waited for a response from the doctor.

Charlene grabbed my arm. Looking to me she said, "When Hilary wasn't crying, my first thought was that she has a heart problem. I'm anxious to know. Does she have a heart problem?"

I could feel Charlene intently tugging on my arm.

Looking directly into Charlene's eyes, I responded, "What would make you think that?"

Charlene replied, "Just a few months after Therese had been born, Connie Ada visited with me. She said that she stopped by to say hello. As we talked, Connie said to me that she once gave birth to a baby that had a serious heart defect and lived for only four hours. When the baby was born, her baby didn't cry."

I responded, "I didn't know. And, I don't feel as if I can interrupt the doctor to find out. We'll have to wait."

As if not hearing me Charlene went on, "And, early during the pregnancy, as you know, I was bigger than I should have been. Shirley Grow, she's a nurse, must have noticed something. During one of the garden club meetings, July or August, she asked me if I wanted a boy or a girl.

"I answered her saying, 'It doesn't matter just so the baby is healthy.'

"At that, she held my hand saying, 'Remember. Special people are blessed with babies that have special needs.'"

As more tears filled Charlene's eyes, as she strained to see what might be going on, she continued, "That surprised me at the time and I didn't think of that until I went to the doctor a month ago. You know I wasn't feeling well as the pregnancy progressed. I looked as if I were expecting twins. I felt I needed to have a thorough check up.

"After the examination, I was sent to the hospital for an X-ray. And, when I returned to the doctor's office, he told me that I was carrying only one baby due in early March."

With a concerned almost desperate look about him, Dr. Earl, coming to where we were, interrupted Charlene saying, "Your baby is not doing well. First indications are that she has a heart murmur. We will need some more time to determine how serious her condition is. I have called for Dr. Harold to come in. He should be here in fifteen minutes or so. In the meantime, we will get the baby cleaned up and we will help her with oxygen."

Charlene and I were dumbfounded. But, we looked at each other conveying a reassurance that eventually everything would be all right.

I thought as I believed Charlene was thinking, "Was Shirley's comment a premonition?"

One of the nurses had placed Hilary in an incubator. Dr. Earl had gone over to check her again.

My mental voice said, "She looks fine. How could something be wrong?"

The second nurse had come over to get Charlene prepared for her recovery. I was asked to go to the waiting room. Though it may have been only a few minutes, time seemed to have slowed down. I became consumed with anxiousness. Moments seemed endless. I paced and prayed.

# 2

On hearing, "You can visit with Charlene," I immediately turned to the door and followed the nurse.

Charlene and I exchanged a smile but deepening concern and anxiety tempered our effort. We had nothing to go on. Something like this had never happened to anyone in our family, relatives included. With the exception of Connie, no one that we knew had a baby with even the slightest problem.

I thought, "How could this be happening to us?"

Again, we reassured each other that everything would be okay even if Hilary had a heart problem.

I said, "They fix hearts and do other amazing things."

Over the underlying concern we shared, we agreed, "Hilary would be fine."

In silence, holding hands, we prayed.

It was almost 1:30 a.m. when Dr. Harold came into the room. He looked tired but offered us a pleasant though concerned smile.

We nodded in reply.

He said, "This is difficult for me to tell you. Your daughter appears to have a serious heart defect and may have other complications as well. Of course, we are not able with our equipment to discern the exact nature of these problems. But, anticipating your approval, a neonatal ambulance has been ordered to transport her to General Hospital. They have the staff and the facilities to evaluate her condition and to take care of her needs. With the bad road conditions, we do not anticipate their arrival for several hours, likely not until late this morning."

Charlene and I looked to each other and then our eyes became fixed upon Dr. Harold.

He added, "The ambulance is well equipped to take care of your daughter even if an emergency should occur en route. Of course, we do not anticipate any difficulties. A neonatalogist is a member of the crew. Your daughter will be in good hands."

"How do we deal with this?" I responded.

Dr. Harold replied, "As time goes on, things will unfold. You will have opportunities to learn more and make the appropriate decisions. In the meantime, be optimistic.

"We will keep your daughter in an incubator with oxygen and we will monitor her vital signs. A nurse will be with her until the neonatal team arrives. Periodically if you like, she can keep you informed throughout the morning and afternoon if necessary. Just try to get some rest. If you need, you may call me. I will be available. And, if I have to, I will come back. The city roads are amenable to travel and I can make it on foot as well."

As we thanked him, at the moment appearing somewhat awkward and perplexed, he took two steps back, smiled again attempting to reassure us, and left the room.

We could do nothing more than wait, hope, and pray.

I sat with Charlene until it was 2:00 a.m. As reported, Hilary was doing okay. Charlene needed to rest and I needed to get home. We exchanged a kiss.

Charlene said, "See you later in the morning. And, be careful going home."

## Hilary Ann – A Broken Heart

As I walked out of her room, somewhat sideways turning toward her as a confirmation that everything would eventually work out all right, I nodded my head saying, "I'll be fine. See you in a little while."

The snow had eased up slightly and the wind had lightened. Just the same, the roads were nearly impassible.

I thought, "If you were able to get to and from the hospital, you will be able to get home. You have a reliable truck and you had managed to negotiate these same roads just hours earlier. So, just get on with it."

On the way, about fifteen minutes later, I realized that Hilary needed to be baptized.

My mental voice said, "You need to turn around."

As I approached the next intersection with a big enough cross section, I let the truck slow down, shifted one gear lower, and spun around making a U-turn. Going back to the hospital was necessary. It was our Faith.

The nurses were surprised to see me. One with a sprite tone of voice said, "Can't you get through? Are you going to be our guest tonight?"

"No," I replied with a little smile and sigh both reflecting my reaction to the nurse and my tired condition. "Nothing like that. I do need a different kind of favor. We're Catholic and I need a priest to baptize our little girl if that's possible. Her name is Hilary Ann."

Without hesitation, the nurse answered, "Sure, if we are unable to get the local priest to come out, we do have a Catholic staff member who has done that before. One way or the other we will take care of that for you."

Nodding my head, I said, "Thank you. And, if Charlene should awake, please tell her."

With a confirming smile, the nurse responded, "Count on it."

Turning, I replied, "See you. I'll be back later."

# 3

Though I had not been able to fall asleep until after 3:30 a.m., I was up at 6:15 a.m. I presumed that Hilary was okay and that her condition had at least remained unchanged.

I called the hospital for verification. The report was guarded.

The blizzard conditions had subsided.

I thought, "Certainly, by mid-morning, the main roads and highways ought to be plowed and the ambulance should be able to get through. In fact, they might even be on their way."

I decided to go back to the hospital. Because I had gotten home well after midnight, Charlene's mother stayed over. She could continue to take care of the girls.

When I walked into Charlene's room, I saw her sitting in bed with a pale pensive stare. In a transparent attempt to be upbeat, I said, "Hello. How are you doing?"

Resonating sadness, anxiousness, and concern, Charlene turned slightly and smiled in a manner that said, "I know you are trying."

I knew what she was saying to me. Words were not necessary. I had the same feelings. I sat at the foot of her bed and began to mirror her expression.

A gentle knock on the door broke into our silence. As both of us focused on the doorway, a cheerful nurse appeared with breakfast for Charlene and as well for me. She smiled in what appeared to be an attempt to raise our spirits. But, we had drifted to where the outside world could not enter. We were enclosed with our fear and apprehension.

Daniel J. Dyman, Ed.D.

We were silent as we picked at our food eating relatively little. From moment to moment, we looked to each other. Our reserved quiet dominated.

My mental voice said, "How do you deal with the unexpected tragedy? Will you be able to measure up to whatever is required?"

I was immersed in uncertainty as never before. I could not tell Charlene because I needed to be supportive and comforting for her. I assumed that she thought about me as I about her.

The moments slowly passed one by one only to be interrupted by another light knock on the door.

Together we responded quickly turning to see who had intruded upon our province of seclusion. Again, it was the cheerful nurse with a pleasant smile. She said, "I can take you to see, Hilary. Would you be ready for that?"

We answered, "Yes. Yes, of course."

It was our first opportunity to see our little girl. She was a pretty little baby, peaceful and appearing to be perfect in every way except that something we could not see was not working correctly within her heart.

I said as a hopeful cheerleader might, "Charlene, we'll get her well. It won't be long and she'll be playing with her sisters."

Charlene was more realistic in her reaction perhaps intuitively knowing that the days ahead would not be easy for us. She looked up to me but smiled cautiously. Then, Charlene turned toward Hilary likely imagining that she was gently and joyously cradled in her arms.

We stood along side the incubator, a baby who we could not touch. Those moments, moments mixed with expectation and

Tears come easy when you are vulnerable, when uncertain, when you are even unsure of hope. I felt that way and I believed that Charlene and I were together equally sharing in the same insecurity.

Signs of weariness appeared on Charlene's face. Slowly we backed away from the incubator not wanting to leave but knowing we had to. Yet, where were we to go? We were not being hurried along or rushed to go. But, we did know that we were about to be handing over our daughter. What could we do otherwise? Everything depended upon someone else. Nonetheless, somehow we had realized that everything depended upon us as well. We paused looking to Hilary wanting and wishing to make everything different needing time to stand still pleading as if it were possible that the moment we were living would in an instant become transformed filled with grandeur and excitement and then remain forever unchanged.

We realized our helplessness.

Slowly, hand in hand, we walked into the maternity waiting room. It was vacant. We sat silently holding hands quietly offering consolation to each other. For the few moments that slipped by, we were in our own inaccessible place isolated in time somewhere in our shattered world.

While we had been visiting with Hilary, Charlene's room had been changed. She was assigned to share a room with Linda Cee who gave birth to a baby boy just shortly after Hilary had been born.

For us the morning was painful. Quietly, seconds merged into minutes. A nurse broke into our conjecture-filled existence at just a few minutes after 11:00 a.m.

She said, "Sorry to interrupt but Mr. and Mrs. Dyman, the ambulance for Hilary arrived moments ago."

We were invited to meet with the neonatal team that would be caring for Hilary. Consent papers had to be signed first by me and then by Charlene. Copies attached to basic information sheets and to a list of protocols for the parents were handed over to me. In addition, we were given a series of verbal assurances that everything would be fine.

The ambulance attendants included a driver, two nurses, and the neonatalogist. Each was dressed in a dark blue jumpsuit ornamented with hospital patches and nametags. They were impressive.

Carefully, Hilary was transferred to a portable incubator and hooked up to the set of monitors that would track her vital signs. We were given an opportunity to see her again but just for a moment.

As Hilary was loaded into the white, orange, and blue transport vehicle with bold red and white lights flashing, we watched through the glass of the emergency room doors.

The doctor and nurses turned to us. We exchanged a wave good-bye. The doors of the ambulance were slammed shut. We were left alone without our child, an empty, helpless, and dreadful moment.

Charlene and I watched for a few minutes as the ambulance with little Hilary drove off winding its way out of the snow covered parking lot and onto the road. Tears began to accumulate faster than they could be wiped away.

Both of us were exhausted. Words were not required. Our attention shifted. We exchanged a hug and a kiss. I left for home. I needed to check on the girls. Charlene's mom needed relief. I needed to call the relatives and friends to let them know of Hilary's birth and the news of her condition. And, Charlene needed to rest.

She returned to her room unaware that she would begin a dear and lasting friendship with Linda.

As Charlene pondered the circumstances, Linda offered support and comfort. In the joy of her new son, she made room for us, especially Charlene. She cried in understanding and offered encouragement. She offered spiritual insights. She reassured Charlene that our loving God would not fail us and that in a special way we were being cared for.

Linda was a God-sent person. After her hospital convalescence, she remained in touch with frequent telephone calls and visits. She was always available for us.

Just after I had left for home, Charlene was surprised by a visit from a church Elder sent by Dr. Harold. He offered heartfelt hopefulness as well as the prayers of his community.

As Charlene introduced him to Linda, Linda realized that she was a member of his congregation. Together, they broke into a delightful laughter over the irony. In coming to visit a stranger in need, an Elder of a church found himself first explaining grief and frustration then joining hands with the presence of joy and gratefulness.

Later that afternoon, Fr. Wright, our parish priest, came to visit Charlene at the beckon of one of our neighbors. His visit would be different from that of the church Elder.

While Fr. Wright had been courteous and extended well wishes, he complained, "If you had your baby in town, I would not have had to go so far especially in this inclement weather."

The circumstances were overwhelming. Perhaps Charlene was overly sensitive but rather than being delighted to serve as she had reason to expect, Fr. Wright appeared overly bothered with the inconvenience he had to endure.

Daniel J. Dyman, Ed.D.

He would give Charlene his blessing but his remarks left her feeling guilty rather than gratified.

While we were not new to the area, we were not well established in town. Only a short time earlier I had accepted a position as instructor of biology and chair of a small rural community college science and mathematics department.

Our second child, Therese had been born in the local in-town hospital. We had not been pleased with the methods of the physician nor the procedures of the hospital. Consequently, we took up an association with a group of doctors in a neighboring town. A colleague recommended the group and we had been especially pleased with Dr. Harold. He had been our connection to Dr. Earl who advertised himself as being "in the practice of obstetrics and gynecology." Later, we would reason that we had gone astray in our thinking. Being, "in the practice of . . ." is quite different from being "board certified in . . ." Perhaps in our lack of attention, Charlene and Hilary had been placed in harm's way.

Early in the pregnancy, Dr. Earl had prescribed an anti-allergy medicine that we later discovered had been linked to heart defects. Would another physician have treated Charlene differently? We will never know. The matter would be haunting.

And, in long overdue reflection, we recalled that just days before Therese had been born, the county highway department sprayed defoliant along the roadways to clear the overhanging tree branches as well as the encroaching bushes. During the first of two episodes in front of our house, Charlene had been in the yard. She felt tiny droplets on her exposed skin, arms, neck, and face. Certainly, she inhaled some of the chemical mist.

As I would discover, the defoliant had been a 50:50 mixture of 2, 4 – dichlorophenoxyacetic acid (2, 4 - D) and 2, 4, 5 – trichlorophenoxyacetic acid (2, 4, 5 - T), simply identified as Agent Orange. We did not make the connection to Hilary's heart defect until well after the Viet Nam war when the findings that eventually were released confirmed the devastating genetic and developmental effects of the substance.

However, in the meantime, with limited insight, after the spraying event, our property had been posted albeit too late, with "Do Not Spray" signs. In addition, I had mailed letters to the editor of several local newspapers in an effort to stop the potentially hazardous spraying everywhere in the county. Some residents frowned, among them one member of the board of trustees where I had been employed. Hopefully with tongue in cheek, but more likely out of indignation, he often referred to me as "the guy who stopped the spraying." Regardless of public sentiment, for one reason or another, the spraying had been discontinued.

# 4

Four hours after Hilary had been taken in the ambulance, a nurse from the Neonatal unit at General Hospital called Charlene to inform her that our little girl had arrived safely, that she was stable, that she would be carefully monitored, and that the neonatalogists and the cardiologists would begin their evaluations the next morning.

For the next ten days, our dealings with Hilary's nurses and doctors had been limited to the telephone. They confirmed that Hilary had a severe pulmonary valvular stenosis, a constriction in the heart valve through which blood passes before going to the lungs. Eventually, she would require surgery.

While we were concerned over the valvular stenosis, the doctors seemed obsessed with Hilary's secondary features, a slight webbing in the back of the neck, somewhat lower positioned ears, and a rather wide spacing between her nipples. Their efforts suggested an unwillingness to accept Hilary as she was. It appeared as if placing Hilary into a known diagnostic category would be the ultimate absolving achievement that once accomplished would provide a clearly certified regimen for her health care.

Hilary appeared normal in all of her other features: toes, fingers, eye position, mouth structure, body proportions, muscle tone, and posture.

The neck webbing suggested that Hilary might have an anomalous chromosome configuration but the karyotype was normal. Tentatively, she had been characterized as a Noonan's syndrome although her features did not qualify her as a "perfect" match. In the course of Hilary's life, this bias would apparently mislead the doctors in their assessments and in prescribing critical treatments.

In the midst of these medical endeavors, Charlene and I had been interrogated about our family history. We had been asked to attend a meeting with a geneticist and we had been expected to participate in the development of a pedigree that might explain Hilary's condition. We had been unable to offer any insights. Simply, our families had no record of any genetic disorders. We perceived that the geneticist was uncomfortable in accepting our truthfulness. Perhaps he thought that we had been deliberately withholding significant information. For our effort, nonetheless, we had been given a copy of Hilary's chromosome profile.

We recognized that we were exceptionally vulnerable and we began to feel culpable as well as graciously devalued.

Stress mounted. We became exhausted. Retribution was due. Over the next several days, it had been exacted.

The third day after Hilary was born, Charlene came home. That evening she developed a deep vein phlebitis that required her to stay in bed with her legs elevated. As an aid, anti-embolism hose had been prescribed. The pharmacist and owner of the local drugstore assured us that the stretchy stockings would be available the next day; however, they did not arrive the next day or the day after that. We called each afternoon for five consecutive days. I presume that the hose never had been ordered. In exasperation, we decided to look elsewhere.

The first telephone call achieved results at another store in a neighboring town, almost eighteen miles away. The hose were ordered and arrived the following day. But now, sick with the flu, in no condition to be gone from home, I had to drive the round trip, a little over one hour. I was not sure that I could be away from home that long feeling weak with a throbbing headache. But, I did make it.

During the drive there and back, I thought, "What is the matter with the local guy? We have an in-town address and telephone number. Surely, he could not have forgotten to place the order for the anti-embolism hose. But, maybe because he did not know us personally, were we presumed to be unreliable, a risk? The hose were not that expensive. Then if we did not purchase them, return them. Get your money back. It would be only an inconvenience. For us the stockings were intended to prevent a life-threatening blood clot. Did he not realize the importance of the prescription?"

If it had not been bad enough that Charlene was off her feet, subsequently, I had succumbed to a more seriously infectious creature. Never before had I become so sick. Venturing away from the bathroom was not an option. Alternating bouts of diarrhea and vomiting kept me busy. At times, I would become extremely weak and perspire so profusely that my underclothing would become soaked. I had been unable to attend the needs of Charlene, Shellie, and Therese. It was pitiful. And, to add to this difficulty, I had committed to lead a four-week interim semester course to research fish behavior in a surface-frozen lake.

I tried to get out of the commitment but the Dean insisted. Finally, he accepted that I would teach only the remaining three of the four scheduled weeks, that under the circumstances, I would do the best that I could. However, that was not an agreement made with one of the students, an ice fisherman enthusiast and the father of one of the college's board members who took the course only for his recreation.

He had been dissatisfied with my performance and anything I did had not been good enough. In desperation, I offered an explanation to the college president, a two-page report on our situation at home and in particular my condition. It had been supported with receipts for prescriptions and records of telephone calls made to our doctor. If it mattered, I was never told. Most likely, it did not. Politics probably prevailed.

I had no rest. Charlene had no rest. Somehow we survived those weeks. Ten days after coming down with the flu and then the incapacitating intestinal disorder and three days into the fish behavior course, I was well enough to at least manage responsibilities of the home and job. Charlene was feeling better and her condition improved enough to permit a visit to the hospital. It was our first break on the daily "Get It Done Today" list. It would be the third opportunity to see Hilary.

Our visit lasted only ten minutes but for the first time, we were able to touch Hilary. The moments were precious. Our visit reinforced our attachment and dedication to our little child and it reinforced our commitment to do everything we could in her behalf.

# 5

Early the next morning Charlene received an unexpected telephone call from a neonatal nurse at General Hospital. She called to inform us that she had been getting Hilary ready to be transported to Pediatric Hospital, a one half-day trip from our home. She assured us that after Hilary became settled someone on the staff of Pediatric Hospital would be in contact with us. No explanation was given for her being moved. We presumed that the time had come for the pending heart surgery that Hilary needed.

At 4:45 p.m., a doctor from Pediatric Hospital called Charlene to inform us that Hilary had arrived safely and that her condition was grave. She said, "Hilary has been diagnosed with meningitis."

Charlene gave the telephone to me. The information was disturbing. The pediatrician tried to overcome my shock with reassurances that with children as Hilary meningitis is not uncommon, that they will immediately start her on antibiotics, and that her prognosis is good.

The doctor added, "Consequently, Hilary's heart surgery will be delayed approximately three weeks to provide enough time for her to fully recover and develop sufficient strength needed to sustain her throughout the surgery time and post operation period.

Also, she said, "Please call anytime for a progress report on Hilary's condition."

Perplexed, I responded, "Forgive me but I do not understand. She seemed well yesterday when we had visited with her. How could this be happening?"

The doctor replied, "With infants as your daughter, dramatic changes can occur in hours. Be assured that we will do our best for her."

I thanked her. We exchanged the customary "goodbye." Then, I hung up the telephone.

My concern was, "Why did the people at General Hospital not tell us that Hilary had an infection and possibly a serious infection? We were there just hours before. They had to have known something was developing."

The next day, late in the afternoon, we received another call from Pediatric Hospital. This doctor informed us that he was the neurologist who had been called in to monitor Hilary and to assist as needed during her recovery from meningitis.

I questioned him about her condition and prognosis. In contrast with the first doctor that had called, he had been reserved about a complete recovery and held open the possibility that Hilary could sustain irreversible neurological dysfunction. He focused on a phrase, "maximize her opportunity," that ultimately tempered every decision that would ever have to be made.

On the fourth day of this hospitalization, Charlene received a telephone call from another staff pediatrician. Initially she asked for permission to take pictures of Hilary because Hilary was covered with an atypical rash that had been linked to the meningitis. Charlene tabled the right of permission until she could discuss the matter with me.

At that point, this doctor queried Charlene, "Why have you not come to visit Hilary?"

Charlene explained our situation. She pointed out that regular classes were about to resume at the college where I was employed and that I was responsible for being there to meet students. She informed the doctor that she had just begun recovering from deep vein phlebitis. Charlene obviously looking for understanding added that we had two young children making travel with them especially difficult because the hospital was over two hundred miles from home allowing only for weekend travel given reasonable weather conditions that at any time could dramatically change causing the development of quite hazardous highways. And, she added that faithfully at least once a day we did make a telephone call for a progress report. In conclusion, Charlene said that given proper care at the hospital, we could offer very little more toward Hilary's recovery.

At that point, the doctor reacted unmercifully, "Well it appears to me that you do not love your baby enough? By not being here for her, you show that you are an unfit mother for this little child who needs your attention."

Perplexed that her explanation to the doctor was unacceptable, Charlene responded defensively, "I assure you that it has not been easy for us. We felt that we were attentive to whatever had been essential for Hilary. And, is not that what you should be doing? Taking care of her!"

The doctor gave no concession and continued her assault on Charlene's presumed lack of concern and disregard with comments that included words as "nonetheless" and "good mothers would be" and "regardless." Then, abruptly she said, "I have better things to do" and hung up the telephone not giving Charlene an opportunity to resolve the issues with which she had been confronted or to even say "Have a nice day."

We would never hear from that doctor again but at the time it had been difficult for us to deal with her barrage of comments. We had been characterized as indifferent toward Hilary while indeed we cared very much about her and her future. We had sufficient stress and at that time, we did not need the burden of any guilt. In addition, Hilary's current illness came about during her stay at General Hospital. We did not bring that about.

Routinely, everyday, morning and evening, we continued to call the hospital for a status report. Each day we were given assurance by one of the nurses that Hilary was progressing well in her recovery. We had been pleased and grateful. And, we persisted in our hope that her recovery would exceed the cautious and conservative prognoses that previously had been offered.

# 6

Finally, the day had arrived for Hilary's heart surgery, twenty-six days from our last visit with her before being transported to Pediatric Hospital. Her ventricular pressure was 126 mm of mercury. We were told that normal would be in the range of fifteen to twenty.

We met with the cardiovascular surgeon, Dr. Edwards. He described the procedure and Hilary's prognosis. We expressed our views on the application of heroic measures to save her already damaged life. He responded with understanding.

Dr. Edwards said, "As your baby, my youngest daughter required open heart surgery. During the surgery, her heart stopped six times. Each time, the surgeon worked desperately to revive her. On the seventh occasion, I told my colleague, 'Enough! All that had been reasonable had been done.' So, I appreciate your desire for a good outcome but respect the need to be judicious in our treatment of your daughter."

Dr. Edwards offered a consoling smile and asked us to be available in the surgery waiting room. It was just after 1:00 p.m.

Charlene and I interrupted our prayers with recollections of every event that took place from the moment of Hilary's birth.

We remembered the nice things that some of our neighbors had done for us. In particular, one of the staff members at the college who on the evening that Charlene came home from the hospital delivered a home cooked meal with all kinds of side dishes and even dessert. Mrs. Fineworth said, "I hope that you will find this acceptable." Did we! It was most thoughtful. The food was absolutely delicious.

I remembered sitting in a special committee meeting only the day before. The college president came in to congratulate another professor on the birth of his eight-pound son. Giving him a pat on the back, he said, "Hell-of-a-man, Doug."

I did try to ignore the moment by looking over the meeting agenda. But, my thoughts shifted to myself and to Hilary, "Was she not good enough for me to merit a congratulatory remark? Except for a few, no one went out of the way to even say, 'I wish you and your family well.' Was I less than a man because I had a daughter who weighed in at just under five and one half pounds and who had a heart defect no less?"

Perhaps the president did not realize his insensitivity and the outcome of his overheard comment. At that moment, I did feel as if I were inferior.

Also, I recalled being stood up by an interim priest on an appointment to discuss the decisions that Charlene and I faced concerning Hilary's pending health care, in particular the heart surgery. I arrived at the church rectory at the agreed upon time. I rang the bell several times. Repeatedly, I knocked on the door. There had been no response. After several moments of standing with anxiousness at first and later with disappointment and dejection, I left feeling as though I had been abandoned.

As I reflected, my mental voice said, "Were you unworthy? Did the priest have an overriding demand that prevented our meeting? Maybe he was justified. When the appointment was set up, he was given a brief overview of the concerns. Was he afraid to offer advice on the matter? But, how will you ever know? You can only wonder as you did then. Later, he never called to reschedule nor did you. The meeting was not fulfilled. Did it matter and would it ultimately matter? As well, you will never know.

## Daniel J. Dyman, Ed.D.

"You needed him before the surgery. Of course, he was taking the place of Fr. Wright who was on a sabbatical leave to study in Rome. How would Fr. Wright have reacted? Nonetheless, if not him, if not the provisional priest, where would you find the dialog, possible insights, and assurances that appeared to be needed?"

The matter of sustaining a vegetative life was a current national topic of debate. Karen Quinlin was burdened with a ventilator that kept her alive while verifiably she had been declared clinically dead. Charlene and I could be facing a similar situation with Hilary. We were concerned about the right decisions to make. What mattered most, a sustained life of unawareness or a brief life totally fulfilled?

With Charlene, I wanted to do what would be right for Hilary. I wanted to maximize Hilary's opportunities but I did not want to put her into irreversible peril. The possibility of such a tragedy tempered every thought and decision I would make with Charlene. I needed to be sure. I needed more than my perspective. That is why I thought a conference with the priest would be helpful.

In addition, I became disturbed because life insurance for Hilary had been denied even after several years of loyalty to the organization that insured everyone in the family. They wrote, "Dear Brother: . . . The preliminary application has been rejected due to medical reasons for Hilary."

My only intent was to provide for Hilary as I had done for the other girls. During the first week after each had been born, I submitted an application for a nominal $2,000 life insurance policy. In my thinking, Hilary was not different from the other girls and she deserved the same as they had received.

After reading the straightforward letter, I thought, "You're not my brother. My brother would not turn away my request even though Hilary had a heart irregularity.

What good are you if you are here for us only when the Sun shines?"

As events unfolded, the insurance would not be needed.

And so, we waited. At 3:42 p.m., Dr. Edwards, still in his operating room attire, appeared in the doorway. With a deep exhaled breath followed by a smile of relief, he softly said, "Everything went well. Hilary is in the recovery room. In a few minutes, you will be able to see her. A nurse will come for you and as days go by, I will be in touch by telephone."

He returned through the door and in moments a nurse took us to see Hilary. The sight of her broke our hearts. Tubes and wires had been attached everywhere on her tiny body. Monitors flashed and beeped. A thick bandage covered her chest and her body was stained with the brown tinge of surgical soap. Only a few minutes were necessary. What could we do?

We made arrangements to call in and check on her status at regular intervals. Our other children needed us as we needed them. We trusted and believed that Hilary's immediate future was reliably in the hands of the hospital's nurses and doctors. Our commitment had been to pray and to be for Hilary as she might have need for us to be. Eventually we would come to realize that only a few individuals including this very special surgeon, Dr. Edwards, were truly caring people as everyone needed to be.

# 7

Hilary recovered more quickly than anticipated. Ten days after the heart surgery she was released from Pediatric Hospital, healthy enough to come home. We were excited. She was fifty-two days old but disappointedly only weighed a scant eight pounds give or take a few ounces.

The round trip took the entire day including nearly two hours at the hospital getting Hilary ready, gathering information to be included in her medical file, signing out, and obtaining medications.

When finally we turned into the driveway leading to our house, we felt blessed. The trip had not been easy especially with our two other children who from time to time needed individual as well as personal attention.

Importantly, we were home looking forward to good days ahead, expecting Hilary to become healthy and grow up with her sisters. We had no clue of all that would take place in the days and months ahead.

In advance, we had set up an appointment to meet with a highly recommended pediatrician, Dr. Erse, who might be more prepared to deal with Hilary's specific needs. Seven days later, she was in his office for a check up. She was a little finicky in eating and a little irritable throughout each day. She had developed a little sniffle.

Of course, she was only two months old and had been through quite a lot. She was not yet nine pounds. We thought that she would gradually get situated with a normal formula and would adjust to the routine personal attention of her mother. The doctor confirmed our thinking and gave Hilary an "all appears satisfactory" on his evaluation.

The next morning Hilary's sniffle turned into congestion. Charlene called Dr. Erse. His response was,

## Hilary Ann – A Broken Heart

"Understand that she is quite small and there isn't much that can be done for her at this point." Through the rest of the afternoon and evening Hilary's condition worsened.

Charlene encouraged me to believe that we could manage. Reluctantly I accepted her effort. Often I was too quick to a conclusion. She was a confirmed mother as I saw her and I had to trust her feelings and sixth sense about Hilary. I convinced myself to be comfortable with her assurances. However, I remained disenchanted with the doctor's response.

I thought, "Surely, some medication must be available that could be prescribed. Something."

I felt as if stuck between the proverbial rock and hard place not wanting to be hasty yet seeing our fragile daughter in distress.

By the next morning, Hilary had developed a temperature. I became very concerned. However, because it was a Saturday, I decided to wait until 9:00 a.m. before calling Dr. Erse. His answering service accepted my call. I persisted in calling every hour until he responded. When we did speak shortly after twelve o'clock noon, he attempted to convince me that really nothing could be done for Hilary at this time.

Dr. Erse said, "Realize that she is less than nine pounds and as I told your wife yesterday there are no medication doses that can be given to a child weighing so little."

I maintained my composure pleading, "Surely, something must be available even for a child as small as Hilary. She had already received an array of antibiotics during her recovery from meningitis."

He replied in a detached tone, "I have other calls to make."

Politely, I thanked him. Inside, I was furious.

I decided to call the primary pediatrician who looked after Hilary at Pediatric Hospital but she was not available. Next, I called, Dr. Harold. As misfortune would have it, he was on a weekend out of town and could not be reached.

With each hour that passed, Hilary's condition appeared to worsen. Throughout the night we were up with her trying to give her nourishment or at least water to keep her from dehydrating. She would have none of it. Her breathing became more rapid and more labored.

The dawn of Sunday finally arrived. Charlene and I were planning to attend Mass each at different times. In this way we could meet our obligations and take care of the girls as well as Hilary. But, about twenty minutes before I intended to leave, about 7:30 a.m., Hilary became cyanotic around the mouth and nose. Suddenly, frustration turned into panic.

I dialed 9-1-1 and explained the situation to the voice that I had heard. An ambulance had been dispatched.

Pickup trucks with blue flashing lights began to arrive in the driveway. Men with no experience in dealing with a situation as this were entering the living room. One by one, four of them arrived. As I could, they were given details of Hilary's condition but none could do anything for her. The ambulance was still fifteen minutes away.

When the ambulance did arrive, the respiratory equipment was quickly brought into the house but it was a mask and valve system for an adult, far too large for Hilary's tiny face. Nonetheless, a technician tried to place the mask over her face.

I shouted, "That won't work."

Puzzled, he looked up to me.

I went on, "She's not even nine pounds. That'll kill her."

Appearing stunned by my outburst, he quickly pulled back.

I calmed down immediately realizing that out of control, I would be useless. Using a suggestive tone, I said to him, "Maybe just hold the mask only near her face so that she might get more oxygen from an enriched but less aggressive environment."

His actions indicated that he understood and agreed. I was pleased.

In a few moments, Hilary's cyanosis began to fade.

I felt relieved but another struggle remained. We had to get the ambulance crew to transport Hilary to General Hospital, out of their range.

Their jurisdiction would only permit them to go to the local in-town hospital. Hilary had never been there. We would have to start at the beginning. Then likely, she would have to be transported by neonatal ambulance to General Hospital. Finally, after some negotiation, only on loan, we were given a small oxygen tank and a mask. We would on our own take Hilary to the hospital.

Thinking about our safety on the highway, I called the state police to be mindful of us providing a description of our van and the roads we would be traveling. Then I called the hospital to give them details and an estimated time of arrival.

Little did we know but this would be the beginning of a routine.

When we arrived, the staff was unprepared to receive us. We had to be seated in the emergency room, had to wait our turn, and then had to repeat every detail of Hilary's history even to the moment. As Hilary fussed dealing with her illness, we had to begin at the beginning while I thought of all of the precious time being consumed as we chronicled dates, doctors, hospitals, and treatments.

My mental voice said, "This should have been expedited. We called ahead for the hospital staff to anticipate our arrival. Could they have at least pulled Hilary's records from her previous visit? This lack of diligence should be reported to someone in charge but who might that be, the doctors, the administrators? Would anyone care?"

In earnest I maintained a cooperative disposition. I would have to adjust to the procedural rules, the ritual of admission. I would have to accept the restricted access to the sanctuary of the medical professionals.

Finally, after many minutes of lost seemingly precious time, Hilary was admitted to the care of the establishment. She had been diagnosed with pneumonia. They took her from us again, presumably placed her into an incubator, and likely initiated an antibiotic regime.

Disclosure had not been of importance. Our uninformed disengaged like it or not acceptance would become all that would ever be needed.

During this hospitalization, we came to realize that our role as parents with responsibilities for Hilary's well-being would be ignored. Increasingly, we came to understand that we were no more than bystanders in her treatment. Our insights, views, and concerns would be of no interest to anyone at the hospital. The doctors and nurses had paramount jobs to perform, requirements to fulfill, and tasks to carry out. Any effort we made to become involved appeared to them to be an encroachment. This exclusion became an ever-present dilemma and an overwhelming hurdle, definitely a barrier to communication.

# 8

Hilary would be hospitalized for an incredibly difficult forty-five days. She would attract a lot of interest under the direction of the doctor team that tended to her during her initial visit at General Hospital. These doctors, Larry, Barney, and Stanley, had assumed overall responsibility for her care. Obviously considering themselves as privileged, they had taken over.

Later, we would discover that this group had been in the loop even while Hilary had been at Pediatric Hospital. During that time, as she recovered from meningitis and the heart surgery, countless other doctors had been called in to attend to her needs and observe her condition. Eventually, Dr. Stanley confided that from the onset he and his colleagues anticipated that Hilary would be back in the hospital and perhaps be back many times.

General Hospital had been only forty-seven miles from our home. We visited Hilary regularly, two times a week and called about her progress when we could not visit. Presumably, because of sound practical reasons but more likely out of pretentiousness, we were sidelined, set aside by the medical staff including the nurses.

We could not obtain insights about her present condition. Our curiosity about how we would manage her future care was of no importance. And, as we quickly discovered, we could offer nothing of value, suggestions or recommendations even about little baby needs. Absolutely, we could make no contribution to Hilary's well-being. Apparently, we were without rightful claims. Our role was relegated to, "stay out of the way" and "do as you are told." We could do little other than pray for her recovery. We did that faithfully.

Daniel J. Dyman, Ed.D.

A little over two months old, weighing in at eight pounds and a few ounces, Hilary had been home with us only nine days.

Generally, Hilary was treated as if she had Noonan's syndrome. However, that never had been confirmed with certainty. It had been a working assumption as is close in the game of horseshoes. She had shown only some of the characteristics. Consequently, we had begun to read all that we could find about this condition. Not much had been known except that individuals such as Hilary had a pulmonary valvular stenosis and a somewhat webbed neck.

Charlene contacted Dr. J. A. Noonan at her office at the University of Kentucky. She had been the researcher who had compiled the list of characteristics of this unusual condition. While she did not express an interest in seeing Hilary, she did offer some supportive and encouraging comments that gave us hope for a placid and reasonably normal future.

Both of us continued to search the literature. Through some investigation and reading, Charlene would discover a group of researchers at a not too distant state medical research center, about five and one half travel hours from our home. She called. They seemed sensitive and genuinely interested. As well, they agreed to meet with us when Hilary would be well enough to travel. We felt fortified with a sense of expectation that kept us going.

We remained vigilant about Hilary's progress. Daily we prayed.

In the meantime, the neonatal doctors had been charting measurements of Hilary's head circumference. It was noted that her head had been enlarging though it had been marginally within the normal range for a child of her age and weight. The watch continued.

## Hilary Ann – A Broken Heart

Later from the medical invoices, we would discover that the neonatal doctors had called in a consulting neurologist to examine Hilary's responsiveness. Apparently, a concern had been circulating about the possibility of hydrocephalus, a consequence of her bout with meningitis. We had not been informed of these proceedings. Later, the reason became ever more clear to us. The doctors were obsessively in charge and they had their own network for involvement. In essence, discounting the input of any outside source including Charlene and myself, they assumed exclusive responsibility for Hilary's total medical treatment but by what right?

Though I reaffirmed my commitment to go on because Hilary needed all that both Charlene and I could give, I chose to block out the possibility that she could develop hydrocephalus.

I thought, "She doesn't need this. How much more could go wrong for her?"

We had hoped that Hilary would be a playmate for Therese. Shellie grew up during my time in graduate school when we had to survive in student housing on only a doctoral fellowship income. Not that Shellie had been deprived in any way but we felt that she would have had a more wholesome environment if she had a sister or brother nearer her age. Because of that, after Therese had been born, we decided to have another child as soon as possible.

Finally, Hilary's condition did improve enough for the doctors to plan her release from the hospital. She had been in the Neonatal unit for thirty-five days. In anticipation, Dr. Larry who was the head of Hilary's pediatric team, called Charlene to inform her of his decision to move Hilary to the Tots ward for a week to ten days before giving her his permission to be released from the hospital.

In her elation, Charlene called me at my office. She began with, "Guess what . . .

I responded with disbelief, "Oh my! That's not right. She's too fragile. I can't believe this."

I hung up the telephone with Charlene and immediately called Dr. Larry. We went over Hilary's condition and his plan.

During the discourse, I encouraged Dr. Larry to reconsider his plan. But, he would have none of my logic. After each of my bits of insight or my pleas to secure his understanding that Hilary was uniquely delicate, he countered with what seemed to be a prepared queue card response reaffirming his mindset, "NO!"

At one point in the conversation, I offered to pay the difference in cost between the Tots ward and the Neonatal unit if space for Hilary remained available.

As much as I persisted, Dr. Larry insisted, "Infants are never released from the Neonatal unit. Around here well babies are released from the Tots ward. If you expect Hilary to be released from General Hospital, she'll be released from Tots. That's final!"

We haggled for nearly thirty minutes. Eventually, I realized my place in this. I had been going nowhere and I would make no progress in getting Dr. Larry to change his thinking. I realized that I was on the verge of aggravating him and that Hilary was still and would likely be for a long time in need of his services.

Without recourse, I submitted saying, "Okay. If you insist, I seem to have no choice but to agree. We'll do this your way."

Politely saying "Good-bye," I hung up the telephone.

During the conversation, I maintained my outward composure and controlled my tone of voice. Inside I was boiling in my frustration.

## Hilary Ann – A Broken Heart

It was Friday just after 2:00 p.m. I was reasonably caught up with my work. I decided to go home. I thought, "After that debate with Dr. Larry, you need a break, a change of pace."

# 9

The next day belonged to Shellie. Later, she would receive her First Holy Communion during the evening Mass. Realization of the intertwined moment about Shellie and Faith enabled me to remain courageous to continue in my obligations beyond any disagreement with Dr. Larry. But, just the same, in my mind, I remained totally convinced that the decision to release Hilary from the Tots ward had been absolutely wrong.

While we should have been looking forward to a party for Shellie, none had been arranged. Except for Charlene's parents, we did not have any nearby family. Consequently, I thought that after the Mass we would have our own impromptu celebration by going to a great little ice cream shop that was only minutes from General Hospital where Hilary had been convalescing.

In my mind, "It was as good as it gets."

We arrived at the ice cream shop just after 9:00 p.m. and in a little less than one hour each of us had our fill of sundaes and tin roofs. As I paid the bill, I asked Charlene and the girls if they would like to visit Hilary. Their eyes sparkled with an unmistakable, "Yes."

Because Hilary was an infant, we had twenty-four hour visiting privileges.

Charlene and I located Hilary's room and walked in to an outrageous surprise. We found Hilary sharing the room with a child in a croup tent who with severe bronchitis had been admitted to the hospital that afternoon.

Instantly, I became upset with the situation but nothing could be done. Hilary had already been exposed and certainly without the approval of a doctor, of course, one was not available who could make the decision, she could not be moved to another room.

My point of view was not to be considered. The charge nurse did not perceive the room arrangement as out of the ordinary. It was a Saturday evening, minutes after 10:00 p.m. She became visibly obstinate. She would not consent to even call a doctor for an opinion. Her final answer was "Absolutely, no!"

The ride home was difficult, indeed. Fortunately, Shellie and Therese were tired and soon fell asleep on a comforter on the floor in the back of the van. Both Charlene and I remained silent. My thoughts were focused on, "How could they have done this? They cannot all be blockheaded but they seem not to have any logic skills."

That Hilary recovered from pneumonia was the only improvement in her condition. Over the last several days, she had gained only one ounce, two at most. And, she was, at least in my mind, vulnerable to any and every infection.

The next morning was Palm Sunday. I was up early with Charlene and the girls. With our Mass obligation already fulfilled, by 9:30 a.m. we drove back to the hospital. I was determined that a room change would be made.

As I walked into the Tots ward, I could feel the tension and uneasiness that my presence brought. Fortunately, an "on-call" physician was available. I was granted permission to talk with him. He had been informed of my concern from the night before and though he had been prepared to meet with me, he could only offer what seemed to be unjustifiable excuses, at best an extremely weak explanation.

From his position seated opposite from me at a round table in the visitor's waiting room, he said, "The child with bronchitis did not present a problem for Hilary. It is very unlikely that his infection could be transmitted to her. He was put into Hilary's room because both children were patients of the same pediatric team. It's that simple."

I responded, "Doesn't anybody here understand how fragile Hilary is? Can they not make associations? Why put her into a risk situation even with the slightest threat? She is a convalescent having had pneumonia and the other child is sick with some kind of acute respiratory infection. It just does not make any sense unless the doctor making rounds wants to save steps during his visitation time."

My remarks were brushed aside as they had been by Dr. Larry the Friday before, as if I were clueless as to what constitutes the essential requirements for prudent care.

Feeling as if I were being placated, treated as an imbecile or a fool, I continued nonetheless, "Undoubtedly, if someone does understand, it appears then that they do not care. Convenience seems to be more important than good sense."

The doctor replied, "I insist that we do care. At worst, maybe an error in discretion had been made. We do not know that your daughter will get sick from this exposure. Realize that she has received a wholesome amount of antibiotics. But, for your satisfaction and trusting that your anxiety would be quenched, I have already reassigned Hilary to a private room."

I answered, "Do you really understand my point of view on all of this? I feel that I had good cause to be concerned. And, the error in judgment as you call it was inexcusable especially after my earlier conversation with Dr. Larry. I pleaded with him not to put her into the Tots ward."

I realized that my last remarks had been unnecessary. He had granted the concession that I had requested. I added, "Thank you for moving Hilary to another room. I do feel better. Thank you."

I stood up from my chair, took Charlene by the arm, and left him. We went to visit with Hilary.

I felt compassion for the nurses who cared for Hilary. Working with her had to be difficult. Typically, she had been uneasy and irritable. At any instant, she could lose her pacifier and would then become exceptionally fussy. And, she would take virtually forever to feed. Her formula had to be thickened with rice cereal so that she could swallow rather than aspirate it. Out of this concern, a special plunger-type system resembling a large hypodermic syringe had been recommended. As needed, it would permit pushing only small amounts of the formula mixture into her mouth.

In the course of our visit, Charlene decided to feed Hilary. With coaxing, it took Hilary over thirty minutes to consume only a couple of ounces likely a maintenance amount of nourishment.

As I watched Charlene, her concern was obvious. I believed that her thoughts were as mine, focused on our little delicate child, "How can we be of help to get you well and to keep you healthy, Hilary?"

We stayed for a while longer watching and praying.

When we arrived at home, Charlene went directly to the linen closet, pulled out a washcloth, and began folding it lengthwise.

I inquired, "What are you doing?"

She answered, "You'll see. I have this idea."

She added two more folds and then folded the wash cloth one more time in half, placed a pacifier in the crease, and secured it with some first aid tape.

Looking up from her accomplishment, she said, "You see, with this wash cloth as a handle, Hilary will be able to better hang on to her pacifier. Let's go give it to her."

I replied, "You want to go back?"

Elated, Charlene said, "Yes, I'm ready. Let's go."

Back in Hilary's room, the pacifier stuck into a folded washcloth proved to be an instant success. Charlene's invention worked.

"You're a genius," I said.

With tears of satisfaction in our eyes, we smiled. Hilary was precious.

# 10

Hilary remained in the hospital for another ten days. We were anxious to have her home but the doctors had become reluctant to give her up. I felt that they were putting off her release because they needed confidence that the incubation time for any possible respiratory infection would have elapsed.

As would become our habit, we visited Hilary every other day and telephoned about her progress when we did not go to see her.

In anticipation of her return home, we purchased a piece of artificial fleece with which to line her crib and car bed as well. We thought that it would make her more comfortable when she slept or rode in the van. As well, we purchased a big white soft and fluffy bear thinking that it would give not only comfort to Hilary but it would provide some support when she would be placed in a more upright position.

We were counting the days.

Finally, the call came, "This is Dr. Stanley. May I speak with Charlene or Daniel?"

Charlene replied, "This is Charlene."

The voice that she heard was business-like, authoritatively straightforward.

"Again, this is Dr. Stanley. I have scheduled Hilary to be released today after 11:00 a.m. Will someone be available to sign her out?"

With delight in her voice, Charlene answered, "Yes, we'll be there at eleven o'clock. Thank you."

Without any scheduled classes, I posted a note indicating that I would be gone for the remainder of the day and without hesitation, I left for home. On the way, I would stop to pick up Shellie from school.

This was a big moment for us. Again, Hilary would be home.

As Charlene and I turned the corner leading into the Tots ward, we immediately noticed Hilary. She was being fed in the hallway next to another child who had just coughed all over her.

"My God," I thought. "How can this be happening? We always show up at the 'wrong' time to discover something else gone awry. Will she ever have a chance?"

Upon looking up, seeing Charlene and me, the nurse quickly took Hilary into her room.

I said to Charlene, "How many times has this gone on without our knowing. Doesn't anybody here comprehend how vulnerable she is? For the sake of convenience or for company, the nurse takes her into the hallway to be fed? Can they not give her a chance? All we can do is file another complaint that does nothing for Hilary and increases the divide. Ultimately, it makes everyone around here think of us as complainers. But, why was she being fed in the hallway alongside another child? She was to have a private room? It makes no sense."

Frustrated as I was, Charlene did not reply. We gathered up Hilary's things. Got copies of her records and charts. Then, at the last moment, as I was about to sign the release, I decided to write a description of the hallway incident we had observed just minutes earlier. It was to be placed in Hilary's file.

## Hilary Ann – A Broken Heart

A few hours later, just as the Sun was setting behind the tree line along our driveway, a welcoming warm glow of light greeted us. We arrived at home, together at last.

We knew that the journey for Hilary would be difficult. But, over the last several weeks, we developed an essential toughness that would give us the strength to cope with adversity and a resilience to endure any hardship along the way.

I assumed that Hilary's welfare was indeed my God given responsibility to be shared only with Charlene and I was determined to never relinquish that for any reason. Somehow by some means we would work to achieve the resources that would be required. I promised myself never to give up and not to quit. Hilary deserved reverence as any other person on earth. In her unique way, she was special. She needed compassion. She was ours to care for.

The next few days were difficult. One or both of us were up with Hilary through most of each of those nights. Charlene accepted the brunt of it because I needed to be at the college alert on the job. We shared time as we could. We talked. We managed.

One imperative on the agenda that needed our attention was the follow-up meeting at the state medical research center, the appointment that Charlene had made two weeks earlier during Hilary's most recent hospitalization.

Two days later we were on our way. The trip there took just less than six hours. While the medical staff was quite accommodating, the outcome was more for their benefit than it had been for Hilary or for us.

From this visit, I recognized the extent of our vulnerability. We had become desperate. Because of our desire to help Hilary, we exposed ourselves to the intrusion of others. We were open to manipulation. For the sake of science, medicine, and mankind, for the sake of benefiting another family in our situation, we permitted a room filled with medical students and associates to examine Hilary and we even gave them permission to take several photographs. I vividly recalled their "hmmms" as they probed her tiny body and measured every feature. The doctors and students saw her indifferently as a learning experience. We saw her as a person with individual merit and worthiness. We were kindly marginalized throughout the examination.

On our way home, disappointment and frustration invaded my thinking. Believing that some kind of remedy must exist not beyond our reach, I continuously thought, "What next? Where do we go from here?"

We maintained our contact with the research center. Periodically, Charlene would call to provide an update on Hilary's condition and progress. We continued to be optimistic that one day, they might give us a helpful insight.

Furthermore, we would begin to feel certain that Hilary's doctors at General Hospital had not been as caring as we thought they ought to be. They were accountable for her during the time when she contracted meningitis. They should have been alert to her particular susceptibility. Clearly they should have known that even the slightest infection could lead to a serious illness. Premature babies are most receptive to infections and accordingly need to be scrupulously cared for. And, on their watch, the hospital staff exposed Hilary to at least two other documented potentially infectious situations.

Later, I would discover that the doctors charted "possible sepsis" for several days before Hilary was finally transported to Pediatric Hospital. On the last two of those days they boldly scrawled "? - *sepsis* - ?" across her chart.

From then on I would ask myself, "Why did the nurses and especially the doctors not respond more expeditiously?"

Charlene broke into my reflective moment. She said, "I've been thinking that we should get in touch with Dr. Henry."

"That sounds fine to me. Call him tomorrow. Set something up. Apart from encouragement, we got nothing from this last group," I answered.

Dr. Henry was Shellie's pediatrician during the time I was in graduate school. He was a fine man as well as a thoughtful and caring physician.

However, we had to postpone this initial attempt for an appointment with Dr. Henry because Hilary came down with a horrid raspy cough the next day after our visit to the research center. For us, this was incredible. Only seven days ago she had been released from the hospital. She had to have been incubating some bug picked up at the hospital, maybe in the hallway during the coughing incident.

The following day we were in the office of Drs. Larry, Barney, and Stanley. After a brief examination, Dr. Stanley prescribed some drops and sent us on our way.

Hilary steadily grew worse. She became increasingly irritable, stopped taking her formula, and struggled to breathe. Her cough became unbearable and she began showing some signs of cyanosis.

Again, it was a Sunday morning. We decided to take her to General Hospital. Because of the previous episode with the local ambulance crew, we had purchased our own oxygen supply should it ever be needed in an emergency. We made our prerequisite calls to the state police and to the hospital.

Nonetheless, when we arrived at the emergency room, all of the details of Hilary's history had to be repeated as if the records in the possession of the hospital system were not immediately available. The questioning would go on and on, "When was she last here? What was her problem? Etc."

I responded, "Everything you will need to know about her history is documented in this folder."

The folder was trivialized. Perhaps expediting admission to the hospital was not as important as I had thought. Perhaps Hilary's records were too much to read. The folder was thick with many pages of documentation. The emergency room physician continued with his questioning and writing of notes. Finally after what seemed to be "forever," Hilary was admitted for treatment.

# 11

At 8:00 a.m., Monday, Charlene called Dr. Stanley to inquire on Hilary's status. He said that he had learned that she had been admitted to the Neonatal unit but he was unprepared to give any details on a diagnosis. He knew that she had been getting antibiotics and intravenous fluids.

Later that morning, just before noon, Dr. Stanley called saying to Charlene, "Hilary appears to have contracted some form of whooping cough. Certainly, she is behaving as if she had contracted some form of infection like that. We have ordered some blood work. Should something definitive come up, I will call you but at any time, you are welcome to check with the nursing staff on her progress."

We were satisfied that Hilary was getting treatment and continued in our anticipation that she would soon get well.

For the record, Hilary's illness would never be diagnosed. All that would ever be charted was "respiratory infection with whooping cough symptoms."

One by one, doctors of every kind were called in to check on Hilary: cardiologists, neurologists, neurosurgeons, and even other pediatricians. Many of them had been consulted from the very beginning. Of course, we were not privileged to know that. Presumably, that was beyond our comprehension level and certainly none of our business.

By this time, word had started to get around the community. Neighbors began to offer their support. We were thankful but with Hilary in the hospital, we were able to manage on our own. Each was given confirmation that if a need should arise, they would be called upon.

The routine continued for us. Every other day or every day as we could get away, we visited Hilary. Charlene would feed her when she could and change her diaper as needed. Sometimes we would just sit with her watching her sleep. Shellie and Therese would wait just outside the Neonatal unit. They were really the most gracious people, somehow understanding that we depended upon their patience even at such an early age.

For two weeks, Hilary remained in her infant bed with alternately either her left or right arm intravenously attached to a jug of nutrients and antibiotics. Whichever arm, it would be the one immobilized with a small sandbag. With the hand of her other arm, she tenaciously held on to her pacifier placed into a folded washcloth as configured by Charlene.

Typically, she was irritable. Her head size remained in the high but normal range. Her heart seemed to be doing fine. At the time, her weight was at just a few ounces over eight pounds. During her hospitalizations, she would lose whatever weight she somehow had gained when at home.

Every visit brought some tears. Observing her struggle for life would at times become overwhelming. Prayers for her recovery filled every moment. Charlene and I sustained a belief that someday, Hilary would overcome the shortfalls of illness. We believed unquestionably that Hilary would eventually grow and develop into a wonderful loving child.

I convinced myself, "As we managed these first four months, we would be there for her the rest of the way whatever it might be."

On the second weekend of her hospitalization, our routine would be no different. After an early Mass on Sunday, we started out for the hospital. This time when we did arrive, Shellie and Therese were asleep in the back of the van. Rather than wake them, Charlene decided to go alone to visit with Hilary.

In minutes, I saw her running across the parking lot toward the van. I became alarmed. I jumped out shouting, "What's the matter?"

When she had reached the van out of breath, she exclaimed, "You should see what they've done to Hilary!"

I woke the girls, picked up Therese in my arms, and hurriedly walked to the Neonatal unit.

Attempting to keep up, Charlene pulled Shellie along. At one point, she shouted, "They've got her all twisted in this baby basket."

As Charlene described her, Hilary was slumped down and over to one side in a baby basket as it might be described that had been positioned at about forty-five degrees up from horizontal. She was seated in an open area on a countertop behind the main desk of the Neonatal unit no doubt so someone could keep an eye on her. In my mind, that was the hospital equivalent to the "one-on-one full time nursing care" that was to be provided for Hilary.

The weight of the sandbag that had been attached to Hilary's left arm had pulled her tiny hand downward almost under the calf of her leg. Her frail body was slouched in such a way that the entire left side of her face with chin slightly upward was pushed up against the left side rail. With her right hand she was grappling with her pacifier.

She was especially delicate and with little muscle tone. The sight of her so positioned slumped and gnarled was deplorable. It was too much for me to observe.

I stopped at the desk immediately in front of where Hilary had been situated, where the nurses and aides were about their activities. Pointing toward Hilary, I demanded, "What is the purpose of this? I need an explanation for what you people have done to this child."

At once the charge nurse looked up toward me obviously not comprehending that something might be questionable if not absolutely wrong. She went on to explain that Hilary began to aspirate her formula and to prevent that from occurring, she had been given orders to place her in a more upright position.

I responded, "Where is her full time care giver? And, what are you feeding her that she has been aspirating it?"

The nurse did not respond to my first question but rather nonchalantly reached over, picked up a small bottle almost filled with formula, and placed it on the counter in front of me saying rather assertively, "This! We give it to her as we can and that's why she's here with us."

I maintained as much composure as I could. We had gone over details many times before. This was too much. I reacted, "This is not her formula. This is some kind of liquid in a bottle. And, where is her feeding device? She requires a formula that is thickened with rice cereal. Everyone here should know that. And, you ought to know that. We left instructions on how to prepare her formula as well as how to feed her with a pump system. It was a routine for weeks. Now, it's changed? Why? What is the reasoning?"

The nurse answered, "Well this is what the doctor ordered for her and I don't know anything about her pump system. Its my first day working in this unit."

"We're going nowhere with this," I retorted in frustration. "We need to get this changed. And, she needs to be lifted out of that outrageous position in that infant basket or whatever you might call it."

The nurse said offhandedly, "I'm sorry, but no one is available who can order that change."

I countered with, "Then, I'll be taking Hilary home with me. Get her things and get her ready to go."

## Hilary Ann – A Broken Heart

The nurse appeared startled. Apparently, she never encountered someone as direct and forthright.

I continued, "Yes, I'm serious about this. If you cannot take care of Hilary as she needs to be cared for, if you cannot properly manage her needs, I will find a place and someone who will care for her. Let's get some new orders written or get her ready to go home. That's it!"

Instantly, without saying a word, the nurse with a startled look turned and hurriedly walked away from me. I remained standing at the desk near Hilary just out of my reach. Within a few minutes, an on-call doctor appeared in the doorway. He asked me to accompany him to an adjoining conference room where we could discuss the matter.

He started with, "You're having a problem?"

I answered, "Yes. As a matter of fact I am having a problem. Hilary's formula had been changed by some arbitrary action and consequently, as reported to me, she had been aspirating it. Does anybody get it? She needs to be on a rice-thickened formula as clearly indicated by the instructions that we had left, instructions that have been ignored. She doesn't need to compound her illness with aspiration pneumonia. You know she was here just a week ago for a respiratory infection. And, you saw how she was positioned in that whatever, baby thingamajig. Is that caring for her or what?"

While I had been on my tirade, the doctor sat without an expression or gesture. He had been tolerant with me in all likelihood repeatedly counting to ten waiting until I would eventually calm down.

But, I continued, "How, can I get you people to do what is required for Hilary? Insurance or not, we are paying a lot of money for her proper care. It appears that she is not getting it."

He answered, "I don't know how all of this came about. I don't know what your difficulties have been and I don't know a lot about Hilary but you can't take her home until she is well enough to go home."

I responded, "Then, please write an order to change the formula as we have it here. Find her nurse. And, please get her out of that contraption into a bed in a private room. Provide the services that this hospital is getting paid for."

I handed over a sheet of paper that Charlene had taken from Hilary's folder that included special instructions for her care as well as all of her medical records.

The doctor examined the sheet of directives and responded, "I think we can do this."

I thanked him but I felt as if I were being conciliated. Again, I felt that all along Hilary had been shortchanged.

Then the doctor arranged for Charlene to mix up some formula and feed Hilary as a demonstration. Lastly, we agreed that he would leave a note that Hilary should not be placed into the baby apparatus as we had found her.

While we felt that we had made an accomplishment, we had only recovered what had already been in place. All of what we settled upon could be undone with the next shift, the next ward clerk, the next charge nurse, the next on-call doctor, or with the return the next morning of any one of her overseeing neonatal doctors.

On weekends, Hilary's doctors were absolutely not available. As we later discovered, one would likely to be out of town while the other two would be presumably at a rest and relaxation hideaway, most likely inaccessible at home.

# 12

Six days went by without a notable incident. Hilary appeared to be recovering. Her white cell count confirmed that. A steady progression into the normal range was being charted.

However, over this time, we became increasingly perplexed because she seemed to have developed a difficulty swallowing her formula even after adding a bit more rice cereal. And, rather than become more peaceful as she did when she had been recovering from an infection, she remained irritable. We were clueless and the doctors were of no help to us because they now had become fixated on her recent respiratory infection. We were left to assume that her newly acquired problem would somehow resolve itself. Generally, we were pleased that she did make some progress in getting well.

Hilary was just over four and one half months old.

We continued our visitation schedule. With each visit, we would bring some fresh clothing and exchange a few small toys. Charlene continued to feed Hilary as she could. We always talked to her and tried to encourage her attention. Again, with each visit, our anxiousness to bring her home only intensified.

When Saturday arrived, we did our usual housework, played with the girls, and decided to attend the evening Mass. We had a good week. I felt that we deserved a treat. I decided to invite Charlene and the girls to visit the little ice cream shop that we had enjoyed before. Instantly, Shellie and Therese became excited. They shouted, "Yeah."

By a few minutes after 9:30 p.m., the girls had delighted in their choice of ice cream served with multiple toppings I presumed all that they could manage.

## Daniel J. Dyman, Ed.D.

As we were leaving, I said, "Is anyone interested in visiting Hilary?"

In unison and without hesitation jumping up and down as only children can, the girls said, "I do."

In a few minutes we would be in the Neonatal unit. Since Hilary had been improving, the doctors, not as before, decided that she should be kept away from other sick children.

As we entered through the doorway of the facility, I noticed that the ward clerk was away from her station and Hilary's private nurse was nowhere in sight. The nurse should have been nearby. Hilary was her only responsibility.

I thought, "Perhaps you didn't notice the nurse because she is in Hilary's room. Or, maybe the nurse could be on an errand."

On entering Hilary's room we found her alone quietly asleep, no ward clerk and no nurse. Her monitors were flashing proper signals. Her heart rhythm and respiration rate were fast but typical for her. We waited for several minutes, neither ward clerk nor nurse showed up.

I began to look about the Neonatal unit area hoping to locate one or the other of them. As my search progressed without finding someone on duty, my concern heightened.

Charlene asked, "What's going on? Is anybody here?"

I responded, "I don't know. But, we need to find someone who is in charge. I cannot imagine that Hilary would be left alone."

While Charlene stayed with Hilary, I continued my search. Several minutes had elapsed after we had arrived. A few steps into the hallway, I noticed a nurse's aid just leaving one of the nearby rooms.

## Hilary Ann – A Broken Heart

I called to her, "Where is everybody? Where's the ward clerk for this unit? Where's Hilary's nurse?"

She answered, "I don't know about the nurse but the ward clerk took a break. She's in the cafeteria."

I thanked her and went back to Hilary's room. I said to Charlene, "The ward clerk is on a break. But, did the nurse show up?"

Charlene answered, "No."

We waited in Hilary's room. About five minutes later, the ward clerk returned. At least seven minutes had gone by from the time I had begun my exploration leading into the hallway, enough time for something fatal to have occurred.

I thought, "How much total time did elapse from when Hilary had been left alone? If needed, who would have been here for her?"

I said to the ward clerk, "Can you tell me where Hilary's nurse is?"

Unaware of my thoughts and feelings, she delightfully responded, "Oh, she left early."

I replied with directness and a somewhat elevated intensity, "Precisely, when?

With a measure of attentiveness, the ward clerk pleasantly answered, "Right at nine thirty."

A bit less aggressive in my approach, I continued my query, "Was she ill?"

"No. It's her husband's birthday. She was to have a party for him," the ward clerk answered now displaying some uneasiness and some concern apparently recognizing the potential for consequences resulting from my initiative.

"Oh," I said. "And, when will her replacement show up?"

Now inclined to be helpful, the ward clerk replied, "She should be here at the shift change. At eleven o'clock."

I chose not to say anymore to the ward clerk. I thanked her and returned to Hilary's room. She may not have been wrong in not having someone cover for her while she went to the cafeteria but the nurse who left early was absolutely out of line. She left Hilary unattended essentially for one and one half hours. In my mind, she should have known better. She needed to be reprimanded.

Seated next to Charlene, leaning toward her so as not to be overheard, I exclaimed but in a hushed voice, "Get this. Without arranging for someone to cover, the nurse went home for a party. Can anyone accept this? It's Unbelievable!"

Charlene answered with a degree of noticeable contempt, "What a place! It doesn't get any better does it?"

Charlene would wait with Hilary until the shift change occurred and Hilary's overnight nurse showed up. I waited in the van as the girls talked and played before falling asleep. After Charlene and I exchanged places, I explained my concern to the nurse who had come on duty and asked her to be in touch with one of the doctors because I intended to meet with whoever would be on assignment the next morning even though it would be a Sunday.

I said, "I'll be here by 10:00 a.m. and I will wait for the doctor as long as may be necessary."

Politely with concurrence, she said, "I'll follow up."

The next day when I arrived at the hospital, a few minutes early, Dr. Stanley was waiting to meet with me. Although I described the events of the night before, his impatient ho-hum mannerisms indicated that already he had been informed of every detail.

When I finished, he looked directly at me as if to intimidate me. He said, "Those are serious charges that you have made."

I responded, "That may be true. Nonetheless, the events I described are accurate in every detail. And, you appear to know that.

"Hilary is an important person in her own right and especially for Charlene and me. She is our responsibility and we are in that sense obligated to do whatever it takes to help her. We pay a lot of money for her care and we feel that we have as many reasons to expect that she will be treated appropriately and properly. So far, we have had some differences about what that might be. I am sure I do not have to recall or go over each in any detail."

He retorted, "You have not been easy to get along with and your actions may be prohibiting the best care that Hilary could receive. Have you considered that?"

Calmly, I answered, "Only because of the series of blunders that the staff of this hospital have made. I rightly took exception to them because of a concern for Hilary's welfare. Now, you are suggesting that in my earnestness I have had an adverse impact on Hilary's care, I caused the entanglements that have arisen along the way. That's outrageous. Which came first, the failures of the hospital staff or my attentiveness to an array of matters that were in fact illogical, inappropriate, and unjustifiable? Which were first, the blunders or the subsequent respective charges as you refer to them? We both know the answer to those two questions.

"The nurse went home early. I did not make that up. I did not cause it. Realize here that I discovered it. A nurse arbitrarily changed Hilary's formula. Another nurse perhaps needing company fed Hilary in the hallway observed there not once but on two separate occasions. A question might be, 'How many other times?' Hilary was assigned to a room with a respiratory distressed child. Then later after our complaints, she was assigned a private room. Why? You know the answer better than I do. These are just some of the obvious shortfalls. How much has happened of which I am not aware?

"Yes, as you say, the charges are serious. Well, repeating myself, the nurse did go home early. That is a matter of record. Her time card should show that. And, we paid for services that evening that Hilary did not receive.

"I trusted the nurse who had left her duties early. I trusted her because of the licensing documents that are posted throughout this hospital."

Not trying to win his admiration, I went on, "Doctor, I have trusted you because of the credentials that you have on the walls in your office. By all of your certificates and diplomas I am led to believe in you and to treat you and your colleagues as if you were at the top of your class but with all honesty, I do not know that. It's an assumption. You or any of your colleagues as well as anyone on this hospital staff could have graduated marginally or at the bottom of their class. From the onset, everyone here had been afforded the highest level of my respect. I assumed that they were the best at what they do. Today, I am not sure about that. I am disappointed at best. That is how it has been for us and especially for Hilary. Would you accept this kind of treatment if Hilary were your daughter?"

At this point, Dr. Stanley was leaning far back in his chair. I knew that he did not want to hear another word.

But, I continued, "Hilary is extremely fragile. Everything needs to go well for her. We have to maximize her opportunity. That is absolutely what I expect. I want to go on from here with confidence. And, that is my intention."

I stood up from the chair and in a polite manner and tone added, "Thank you for listening. I know my way out."

Dr. Stanley did not respond. As I left, I felt justified. I wondered what impact my remarks would have. At that moment, it almost did not matter.

I saw the situation, no doubt differently than the medical staff. Hilary needed to be protected. She needed all of the care that had been directly or indirectly agreed upon, reasonably the minimum of what might be defined as considerate care and as rightly could be assumed.

In accepting Hilary into the hospital, we were given a certain assurance. And, in accepting payment for services, though from a third party insuring agency yet supplemented with my checkbook, that commitment was at least reasonably guaranteed. The unwarranted had not been demanded. Rather, it was caring that was due and expected proportionate to the true worth and value that is inherent in every individual including Hilary.

# 13

I recognized that the way our relationship had been going with the doctors and the hospital staff that we desperately needed to find another pediatric group to care for Hilary when eventually she would be released from the hospital.

Her release could not come soon enough. Twenty-seven days after being admitted for some undiagnosed whooping cough-like illness she was discharged directly from the Neonatal unit. This time we did not have to suffer through the Tots ward program. The issue had never come up. Perhaps a new wrinkle had been added to the medical repertoire. We were grateful to have Hilary at home.

Hilary was one week short of being five months old. She had been hospitalized for all but nineteen days. She had gone through more than most people ever experience in a lifetime. Remarkably, she still weighed just a few ounces over eight pounds.

With her release came the instructions to administer a postural drainage procedure to keep her lungs clear. Three times a day, her back had to be thumped while her body was elevated above the level of her head. That had to have been awful for Hilary. Had she the ability, in all likelihood she would have screamed, "Stop! With your therapy, you are causing an unbearable head-throbbing pain."

It was not anything we wanted to do but the treatment was administered faithfully.

We again connected with Dr. Henry, set up an appointment, and drove most of a day to visit with him.

He was delighted to see Shellie again and was pleased to meet Therese.

## Hilary Ann – A Broken Heart

After the exchange of various recollections and pleasantries, he examined Hilary but offered little by way of insight.

He encouraged us to continue what we had been doing and supported the idea that we should trust our intuition about what to do for our stricken little child. Before leaving, he gave us the name of a nearby but out-of-state pediatrician whom he thought might be helpful should the need arise.

The trip home was quiet. Silence prevailed.

We got less than we had wished for but not more than realistically we had anticipated. Hilary was not doing well and we were becoming more and more cautious about her future. We encouraged ourselves to hold on to our beliefs and we persisted in cultivating an optimistic outlook. Hilary needed our positive disposition. Though she could not say it, she needed for us to be all that we could be for her. And, in some inexplicable way we needed her so very much.

Each day that she was with us, Shellie and Therese seemed to grow closer to each other and to Hilary. They would stand side by side with Charlene when she would tend to Hilary. They would sit next to Hilary and they would quietly watch her sleep. They would carefully touch her, lightly pat her back or shoulder, and gently would hug her whenever they could. From time to time, Shellie would hold her in her lap.

Again, Hilary appeared to be making progress. Again, we recovered our hopefulness.

We developed a charting system to keep what we thought might be essential data. The chart included the amount of formula and water she consumed as well as her daily weight, head circumference measurements, and notes about her disposition, calm or irritable.

Next, we set up weekly appointments with Dr. Stanley and at one meeting we offered our data. He responded as if amused by it all but we persisted trusting in the importance of our effort.

Hilary had gained some weight. From day to day it tended to fluctuate an ounce more or less. She was approaching nine pounds. The thought that she was getting to be a heavyweight made us smile a bit.

Her head size increased a little but still remained within the normal range. We supposed that as with developing infants her head was developing more rapidly than her body but eventually her body proportionately would catch up.

She remained irritable. Sometimes she would become tense tightening every muscle it seemed. For those moments, we had gotten a prescribed sedative medicine. The occasional few drops would quiet her. We were becoming used to Hilary.

Thirty days after being released from the hospital, a little over five months old, we took Hilary to Pediatric Hospital for an auditory checkup. Charlene felt that Hilary might have a hearing problem as a consequence of the meningitis. She did not appear to respond to voices or to the sounds of musical toys. The results of the testing were conditional but her hearing as well as could be determined was considered normal. For us, that was another positive as was each day that she remained healthy and home with us.

Another month had passed. Our weekly-visit-to-the-doctor program began to deteriorate. Hilary became more irritable and she became tense stiffening her body more frequently. Occasionally she refused to take her formula. And, sometimes when she did take her formula she would throw up. This too began to occur more frequently as did our telephone calls to the pediatricians.

## Hilary Ann – A Broken Heart

When Hilary would become too difficult, Charlene would call Dr. Stanley or one of his colleagues whoever was available in the office. As we kept trying, we apparently became more tiring for Hilary's doctor team. They were losing patience with us and as might be expected, Charlene had become increasingly intimidated by them. She became reluctant to call. However, I encouraged her to continue.

During the stress moments that occurred, I would say to Charlene, "Hilary needs your effort and persistence. Don't let them put you off."

Separately, I spoke with the doctors as to how we might deal with Hilary and her difficulties. Three times we set up a plan that would fall apart in maybe hours certainly in just a few days. Apparently, essential communication among the doctors did not take place. We needed the continuity that was apparently absent.

The pediatricians continued their rotation system of being away from the office. One would cover for the other two. Over weekends a substitute would be on call. No doubt Hilary's doctors were trying to stay fresh in their work but alternating with them was difficult for us in our situation. Consequently, the more we tried, the more they grew weary of us.

I thought, "If not to you guys, where do we go with Hilary? You are all she has."

Hilary was in the sixth day of her seventh month when she again refused to eat. This time she persisted for three days. Hour after hour even throughout the night Charlene tried to get her to take some of her formula. With each effort, Hilary spit it out. She appeared to be dehydrating. When gently pinched, her skin showed only a slight sign of resiliency. With concern, Charlene called the doctors. Only Dr. Barney was in and with the telltale sign of reluctance in his response agreed to see Hilary. After a hurried trip, speeding as I could ten to fifteen miles per hour over the limit even in city traffic, we arrived at the end of the day, just minutes after 4:00 p.m.

Charlene described the situation for him. He said nothing. He walked out of the examination room and in a few minutes returned with a bottle of some kind of formula. He took Hilary into his arms, put the bottle into her mouth and she began to frantically suck it down.

Charlene and I were flabbergasted.

Dr. Barney looked up at Charlene and said, "Try to do the same thing."

I felt that his comment was uncalled for and reacted contemptuously, "You don't know how much we have tried but since you are so good at this, you keep her."

I took Charlene by the hand and proceeded to the door. As I reached for the door handle Dr. Barney responded, "You can't leave her here."

I answered, "You're right. I know. I was only kidding. I wouldn't think of leaving her with you."

Appearing startled, he responded, "You know, you're always calling at the end of the day or during the weekend."

I replied, "Is that what's bothering you? It may appear to you that we wait to call only late in the day or on weekends so as to inconvenience you but we call only after we have struggled through the day and night and even through the weekend. Working with Hilary has not been easy.

"As just a moment ago, you didn't have to treat Charlene as you did saying to her 'Try to do the same thing.'

"She has given everything she has in helping Hilary. You have no idea how much.

## Hilary Ann – A Broken Heart

"Your assumption of us is incorrect. You talk down to us as if we are incompetent. As a few days ago explaining to us that Hilary has blue blood flowing into her heart and red blood flowing out. We know quite clearly the events in the circulation of blood.

"You appear to see us as annoying and unreasonable as today when you complained about the time when Charlene called.

"Let me assure you that we are conscientious and knowledgeable. I have an earned doctorate as you do. You know that. My specialization was in cellular and molecular biology coupled with education. From my perspective, you have no corner on intelligence. The only difference between us is the area in which we did our work and the responsibilities we have taken on.

"Furthermore, when we have on occasion sat down to draft a plan, typically it would fall apart in no time at all. We were not the ones who were unavailable or out of town. We trusted in you or someone fully informed to be available for Hilary. I want you to understand that and we feel that you have not always been here for her when she needed you. In addition, you appear to want us to be submissive. Why can't we be collaborative in this?"

Dr. Barney interjected, "We do try. And, we are concerned for Hilary's welfare."

"Thank you," I answered. "I'm gland to hear that. But, I would truly like to believe it."

I continued, "However, apart from everything else, may I ask you the name of the formula? We will gladly use it if that is what she will take."

Dr. Barney gently returned Hilary to Charlene's arms saying, "Excuse me. It is a sample but I will get the can."

Daniel J. Dyman, Ed.D.

We seemed to have reached a new plateau in our relationship. I felt pleased and Charlene looked somewhat relieved. She does not like it when I push a point but I believe that on some occasions, a person has to be straightforward to achieve a needed understanding.

In a few moments, Dr. Barney returned. He handed over to Charlene a sample can of formula. He seemed pleased to have done that. Together, we thanked him.

On our way home, we stopped at a supermarket to buy some of the new formula for Hilary.

# 14

Four days later, Charlene received a telephone call. The person was angry. After being assured that he was speaking to Hilary's mother, he curtly said, "Where have you been? I expected to see Hilary six weeks ago."

Charlene stammered, "What about six weeks ago?"

He responded as if frustrated by the question, "I left instructions for you to bring your daughter in for a check up when she was six months old. I want to know why you did not follow up?"

Charlene answered, "We did not follow up because we did not know you wanted to see her."

He replied adamantly, "I left word with her doctors at General Hospital. Didn't they tell you?"

Charlene answered, "No one told us anything. And, if I may ask, who are you?"

Apparently taken by surprise, his tone somewhat moderated, he responded, "Who am I? You don't know? I'm the neurologist that looked after Hilary when she was at Pediatric Hospital with meningitis? I'm Dr. Noah. How is your daughter?"

Charlene responded, "As you now may realize, we were not informed of your request. And, as for Hilary, she is getting along but lately, not too well."

Apparently appeased, in a calm encouraging tone of voice, Dr. Noah replied, "I want to check up on her. We can discuss the details then. I want you to make an appointment with my receptionist and I will look forward to seeing Hilary. Let me transfer you."

Daniel J. Dyman, Ed.D.

The telephone clicked. A moment later, an appointment was arranged, set for September 3, three days short of when Hilary would be eight months old, the day after Shellie's seventh birthday and just about two weeks before Therese's second birthday.

When Charlene told me of Dr. Noah's telephone call, it was obvious that Drs. Larry, Barney, and Stanley intentionally withheld from us his interest in Hilary.

I said, "They just didn't forget to tell us, Charlene. Do you recall? From time to time, they have had their associate neurologist looking in on Hilary."

Charlene asked, "What could be their motives?"

I responded, "Please. I have no idea. But in this matter as in others, they have not been forthright with us."

We were disappointed and we became more convinced that we needed another pediatric group for Hilary. I looked forward to the appointment with Dr. Noah believing that something good would come out of our meeting. Since Dr. Edwards, he was the first to show a somewhat sincere concern for Hilary's welfare. On his own, he had called to follow up and to inquire.

Hilary remained unsettled. The postural drainage routine continued. We kept our chart that literally showed no improvement over the past several days. Hilary did not gain an ounce. Her head circumference increased a few millimeters. She continued with bouts of not eating and throwing up. We struggled.

The day arrived to meet with Dr. Noah. We gathered in the waiting room, about fifteen minutes early. The reception area was unexpectedly huge. It was painted white with pictures of scenery periodically placed to interrupt the monotony. Several straight-backed modestly cushioned chairs had been methodically spaced along the walls. Small

## Hilary Ann – A Broken Heart

tables with a few stacked magazines had been positioned between every other chair. The atmosphere was aseptic, indisputably cool. On either end of the wall opposite the entrance was a door each with an adjoining small sliding glass window. A bell button was positioned between the respective doors and the windows. It was through the small window that we would be signed in.

Crossing the room, I proceeded to the window to my left. I pushed the button. In a moment, the window opened. I announced that we had arrived with Hilary. Cordially, I was given a clipboard and a form to complete. It requested the usual first time visit information: name, address, who to contact, insurer, nature of the problem, etc.

In a few minutes, with Charlene's help I completed the document and returned it through the window. Hilary was quietly resting on Charlene's lap. Shellie and Therese sitting next to me were leaning one on each arm tired from the long morning drive. We were all tired.

The door next to the small window suddenly pulled open. We were startled by it. A bright looking woman perhaps in her mid thirties dressed in a white outfit trimmed with an olive green piping around the collar and cuffs approached Charlene, smiled and said, "My name is Gail. May I have Hilary?"

Charlene got up as if to go with her but the woman reacted, "No, no, I just need the baby."

Charlene with Hilary in her arms stood still not sure what to do.

Remaining seated, looking up, I said to the woman wanting to take Hilary, "Charlene can go with you."

Seemingly unsettled, she responded, "No, just the baby."

I replied, "But we are not used to that. For us it has been customary that wherever Hilary goes her mother goes."

With a rather flip tone of voice, the woman responded, "Well, today that will be different."

I stood up shaking my head from side to side and said, "Well, in that case, we wasted our time coming here."

I turned to Charlene saying, "Let's go."

The woman reacted as if seeking understanding, "The examination room is quite small. There isn't enough room for the baby and mother."

I answered, "Charlene won't take up much space. She'll stand in a corner where she's out of the way."

The woman again insisted on taking Hilary without Charlene. To that I turned, took Charlene by the arm, and nudged her toward the exit.

On taking one step, the woman said, "Okay, if you insist, she can come, too."

With a look back I said, "I appreciate that. Thank you."

As the woman then turned to lead the way, I said to Charlene, "We'll be in the van."

Charlene with Hilary followed through the doorway. Shellie, Therese, and I slowly walked to the van. They needed to rest.

In minutes, I saw Charlene hurrying toward the van.

I thought, "Oh, not another episode."

Charlene pulled the passenger side door open and said, "I need Hilary's sedative drops."

## Hilary Ann – A Broken Heart

She reached behind the seat and pulled the small bottle from the travel bag. Without hesitation, she turned, pushed the door shut, and ran back to the building. I moved my seat back as far as it would go to get comfortable and to relax. The girls snuggled in their sleeping bags.

The next I heard was Charlene screaming, "They won't let me back in."

I jumped up, woke the girls, and I carrying Therese and Charlene pulling Shellie ran to the doctor's office. Indeed, it was another incident.

When I arrived in the waiting room, I let Therese slip from my arms standing her on the floor. I went up to the small window, slid it open, stuck my head in to see the receptionist an arm's length away and emphatically said, "I want Hilary. I want our baby returned to her mother."

Startled, she looked up.

Again I said with more emphasis on each word, "I want Hilary! You have taken her from her mother. I want her back, immediately!"

Without a word, the receptionist got up, twirled around, and quickly disappeared through a side doorway. I was locked out. Breathing deeply, I waited.

Thoughts rushed through my head, "They kidnapped Hilary. But, if I called the police, I would be the one in jail tonight. He's the doctor. I'm just the patient's father, the nothing, the one always to be dealt with, the one to be pleading and submissive."

Dr. Noah appeared in the window bending down slightly. Seeing me, he said, "What's the matter? What can I do for you?"

I replied, "I want Hilary back. The woman who identified herself as Gail, presumably your employee, now with our baby, locked Charlene out."

Dr. Noah responded pleasantly, "Come in. Let's sit and talk about this."

He stood back and then pulled open the door next to the window. I entered with Charlene.

Pointing to Charlene, I definitively said to Dr. Noah, "She needs to be with Hilary."

Dr. Noah answered calmly in a quiet voice as if to control me, "We may do that but let's take a moment. Let's go to my office and talk about this."

We entered his office. As we walked in, he positioned me in front of a colossal leather chair and then gave me a shove into the chest so that I fell backward into it. It was extremely soft. I felt as if I had slipped through a cloud almost to the floor.

Now, standing over me, pointing to me, and posturing, Dr. Noah in a dominating tone said, "We are having a problem here. Are we not?"

I heard the reference to "a problem" once before. I thought, "This has to be a conditioned response in all likelihood learned in a medical school psychology class, a technique for gaining control and diffusing an altercation."

Before Dr. Noah could go on, I pushed myself up from the chair to stand on his eye level and interjected, "Yes we are having a problem here as you say. You requested this visit. We came. Our custom is that Charlene is with Hilary wherever she goes.

"She had been permitted to accompany Hilary at the onset of the evaluation or whatever the procedures were to be but then she had been misled and subsequently locked out. That's why I'm here and unless Charlene can go into the examination room with Hilary, I want Hilary back and we're leaving. I didn't come here for a contest."

Dr. Noah said, "I understand. Please sit down. Wait for me to make the arrangement so that Charlene can be in the room with Hilary."

Charlene followed him. I continued to stand. When he returned, I explained that Shellie and Therese were tired from the long ride and that they needed to get some rest in the van. I excused myself to avoid any additional confrontation.

An hour later, Charlene was at the van with Hilary in her arms. I opened the door. Charlene placed Hilary in her car bed and began to go over the remainder of the schedule.

Because Dr. Noah's other machine, the one for the brain scan was not working properly, we were directed to go to a laboratory across town to have that done. The EEG (electroencephalogram) part of the examination along with undisclosed ancillary tests had been completed. The details and findings of these only referred to assessments were never discussed with us. They took place during the time that Charlene was led on a wile and out of the examination room.

On the way, Charlene said, "The nurse lied about the examination room. It was not a ballroom but it was big enough for ten people to be in there. And, when I was let back into the room, Hilary was tied up to a board and already asleep from whatever she had been given. That woman did not need the sedative drops as she said. That was her ploy to get me out of the room."

I reacted, "I know. How clever. And, I am really angry about that shenanigan. Why must these medical people always have to be so condescending and possessive even secretive about what they do? I had thought that Dr. Noah was truly interested in Hilary. I'm having second thoughts."

The girls were lying on the floor in the back of the van. Hilary was asleep in her car bed. Charlene pushed back in her seat appearing exhausted from the stress. Following the detailed directions, I drove to the given location for the prescribed brain scan. We arrived thirty minutes later. Charlene managed with Hilary. I stayed in the van with Shellie and Therese. At the moment they were coloring pictures.

In a few minutes short of one hour, Charlene with Hilary was opening the door. When she got in and before she could put Hilary into her car bed she began, "Guess what!"

I answered, "I can't. Tell me."

Charlene continued, "Well, he did some scans of Hilary's head, I have the pictures here, and the technician said that in Dr. Noah's office, Hilary was given chlorohydrate, essentially a Mickey Finn. He said that we should have been told to keep her alert because she could go into a coma. Great, huh? We're driving along. She's sleeping. How were we supposed to know? That woman, Gail, didn't tell us! That makes me doubly angry."

And, I became angry as well. Frustrated, I answered, "I can't explain it, Charlene. No matter what we have done, someone is always in the way doing something to cancel out any progress or potential progress. But, as long as Hilary is ours, I'm going to do what I would consider to be right for her. Do you agree?"

Charlene answered, "We don't have a choice in this. There's nothing else."

When again we arrived at Dr. Noah's office, I announced our return and within a few minutes Dr. Noah eagerly opened the door and greeted us cheerfully with a smile as if all that earlier had transpired had been forgotten. I was undaunted by his gesture of courtesy. I had other things on my mind all related to the treatment of Hilary. I made an effort to be calm and composed to see where all of this make-believe was going.

Appearing anxious, one hand clasped by the other at chest level, Dr. Noah said, "Do you have the pictures?"

I answered, "Yes, they are here in this envelope. However, I do not want to give them to you until I am assured that you will be forthright with me about everything that concerns Hilary. And, I need to know that you will give me a copy of everything so that I can include it in Hilary's personal file. We keep her records wherever we go."

Dr. Noah appeared set back by my directness. Perhaps no one had ever spoken to him in that manner. However, I had become worn out with the maneuvering and the continuum of deficiencies, impediments and failures that we had encountered in trying to do our best for Hilary.

Caring for Hilary was a serious business. Her well-being was in the balance. Still one blunder one mistake after another curtailed our every effort to help Hilary become all that she could have been had she not gotten a hospital associated illness in the first place. She had been at the mercy of countless people and until now only one doctor absolutely understood. That was the cardiovascular surgeon and perhaps he understood only because he had a child that died as a result of a congenital heart defect.

Dr. Noah led us to his office. Surprisingly, he responded with a measure of understanding and sincerity. He generalized telling us that Hilary did not respond properly to all of the tests performed by his technician and that Hilary's EEG was bothersome. Some of her brain waves were peculiar.

Daniel J. Dyman, Ed.D.

I handed over the coveted photos. The brain scan was as suspected. Hilary needed a shunt. We would need to find a neurosurgeon in our area. Scar tissue from the meningitis restricted the passageway for cerebrospinal fluid to leave the brain. The fluid had been accumulating in the cerebral ventricles. Hilary was in the early stages of hydrocephalus.

# 15

Ultimately, Dr. Noah was compassionate and gracious. He helped us find a neurosurgeon for Hilary. He wrote a lengthy letter of introduction together with Hilary's medical history, as he knew it. It included every detail of his involvement. He had to have understood my feelings of custody and responsibility for Hilary.

It would be seventeen days before we could meet with the neurosurgeon. In the meantime we celebrated the birthdays of both, Shellie and Therese. They were gala affairs, fun for each with cake, games, and lots of giggling. Friends and neighborhood playmates were invited.

As we drove to meet this doctor, we realized that we could not go back in time. We realized that we had been trying to overcome an obstacle that would likely continue as a barrier. We realized that we were still trying to accomplish a participative working relationship with the doctors, especially Hilary's neonatal pediatricians. It had not happened and probably would not happen. We agreed that a positive working relationship was the correct approach in helping Hilary. We would have to make that clear.

We did not want confrontation with the doctors. We did not want to do their work. Hilary was our responsibility. We were liable for her, to speak in her behalf, to choose from among alternatives that were available. We needed information. We needed to understand the options. As parents, we needed to make the decisions that affected her life.

Of course, when we sensed that she had been neglected or found that she was in any way receiving less than her entitlement, we were compelled to let that be known. We would have been remiss had we not responded. From the onset, we encountered enough shortfalls in services rendered justifying all of our reactions. These were appropriate. In time, we had grown at least cautious as a result and perhaps too distrusting and over protective. Sincerely, we felt that we had no other recourse.

Hilary's care was complicated. Rightfully, no one had a clear and precise plan or even the proximity of a program by which to proceed. So, why not be open about it? Children with complications do not come along often and they are not all alike. Dr. Harold understood that immediately. After Hilary's heart surgery, we approached him to serve as her primary care pediatrician. He declined because he felt under prepared for her. He did remain our resource for Shellie and Therese through their early teen years. We had always thought of him as a friend and ally.

We were being drained of our energy and strained in our hope. Somehow through fate, Hilary was assigned to us as had been Shellie and Therese and we to them. We had to go on. We had to be for each girl as would be needed. We had been given the means until now and we were convinced that these resources would sustain us through whatever was ahead.

We arrived at the office of the neurosurgeon, Dr. David. He read our letter of introduction and reviewed Hilary's medical history especially the materials from Dr. Noah. He physically examined Hilary and in detail described the nature of the anticipated surgery as well as the purpose and function of the shunt. Straight up, he asked us if he should proceed. His candidness was convincing. He had been highly recommended.

We agreed. We felt that for Hilary's benefit, the only prudent option was to go ahead. In some states, surgery to "correct" the complications of hydrocephalus was mandated.

The neurosurgeon responded, "Realize that I am not God but you can expect that I will do my best."

I answered, "That's all we ask for, your best effort."

We explained some of our experience in caring for Hilary and inquired if the surgery could be done somewhere other than General Hospital. His solution was for her to be at Community Hospital, conveniently a few blocks away from his office though a little farther from our home. He suggested that we visit there and meet the people who would be caring for Hilary.

En route, I thought about Dr. David's exclamation, "Realize that I am not God . . ." Truthfully, we did not expect him to be God. Ideally, we only needed him to be helpful and caring."

The surgery was scheduled to take place in four days, on September 24.

It became apparent to us. We understood why Hilary was refusing her food and why when she did eat, she would frequently vomit. The pressure from the accumulation of cerebrospinal fluid in her brain was causing her stress and her intensified irritability. And, our effort in postural drainage only exasperated the pressure. With the doctors suspecting hydrocephalus, that given the most understanding, had been truly bad advice.

"My God," I thought. "On that highly regarded recommendation, what were we doing to her?"

I realized that we had to go on. We had to continue. In four days, her stress would be alleviated.

On the way to Community Hospital, Charlene said, "Things may be working out for Hilary."

I answered, "Let's just hope that this hospital is acceptable."

Charlene replied, "I'm glad that we were able to have Hilary officially baptized last Sunday. At least if something happens . . ."

I interrupted, "Charlene, we're on our way to take a look at this hospital. I agree with the baptism. How could I not? But, nothing is going to happen to Hilary. Let's be positive. She will make it and she will get better. I feel good about Dr. David."

Charlene answered, "I know. I understand."

The formal baptism took place at Our Lady of Consolation Church where Fr. Lou was the pastor. He was a longtime family friend and administered the sacrament. The Godparents were special to us, Nancy Bea, a niece, and Felix Kay, an uncle through marriage.

Hilary was chosen as the name out of admiration of a former student, one who was bright-eyed and cheerful in her ways. The sound of the name gave us a sense of joy and we trusted that Hilary would be pleased with our selection. Later we would discover that Saint Hilary is the patron of developmentally challenged children. With that awareness, her name seemed to have been assigned providentially. Ann was selected as it had been for Shellie and Therese, to honor the mother of Mary, the First Lady of the Church.

We walked into the lobby of Community Hospital. From there we were directed to the fourth floor where we met Ms. Susan, the head of the pediatrics department. She explained that they did not have a neonatal unit for special care situations as Hilary's but she did say, "Nonetheless, we feel comfortable with the management of her care given our facilities."

In her approach, she gave us confidence. She made us feel at ease. Her comforting disposition gave to us yet another occasion for renewed hope. We thanked her for her time and expressed our appreciation. Again, Charlene and I felt positive about Hilary's future.

# 16

Hilary's surgery to install the shunt went well. We were permitted to see her after being released from recovery. Her head was bandaged. She looked as if she were in a stocking cap. She was so very delicate, so very precious.

An outline of the tube beginning in her brain that ended in her abdomen where excess cerebrospinal fluid was to be reabsorbed and recombined with her blood was observable passing under the skin of her neck. The small regulating valve placed under the skin behind her right ear was also apparent. With shoulder length hair, none of the apparatus would be noticeable.

Her progress after surgery was remarkably quick. That confirmed our revitalized hopefulness.

The nurses of Community Hospital who cared for Hilary were special. From our experience, she was difficult to manage yet some of them specifically asked to care for her. They really liked her. That was obvious, unexpected, and consoling.

In the background, pediatricians and cardiologists checked on Hilary. They were with a different group. That was also surprising and good.

Eleven days after the surgery, approximately nine months old, weighing in at only eight pounds and eleven ounces, Hilary was released from the hospital.

Again, she would be home with us. We were happy and looking forward to better days.

We were instructed in how to operate the shunt valves but we were uncertain about problems if they were to arise.

Hilary's neurosurgeon assured Charlene saying, "Mother's know when something is wrong. You'll know."

Nonetheless, we did not have the confidence that he presumed. Our past experiences may well have dampened that perspective.

Gradually, life for us began to return to normal and we became less dependent upon Drs. Larry, Barney, and Stanley. We did take Hilary in to the neurosurgeon for a weekly check up. In addition, she regularly visited her cardiologist. She was doing fine.

The shunt was working properly. Hilary seemed to be more relaxed and considerably less fussy. She had even gained some weight. Postural drainage was an event of the past. An overall calm had developed. Her progress continued for over two months.

However, in early December, Hilary became increasingly irritable. The shunt had begun to fail. On December 6, when she was exactly eleven months old, the valve had to be replaced. This time, her progress in recovery was slower than before.

Christmas was not a happy time for us. Our family was incomplete but we did what we could for Shellie and Therese. Santa did come to visit leaving a bounty of gifts under the tree.

Twenty-two days after the revision, on December 30, another revision was required. The drain tube needed to be replaced.

Seven days later, Hilary "celebrated" her first birthday while in the hospital.

The nurses brought birthday cards and several balloons. With them, they decorated Hilary's room and bed. And, they presented her with a "Happy First Birthday" cake even with a candle and invited other children from the ward to attend her little party. They sang, "Happy Birthday."

Though it was thoughtful, something nice that someone did for another, and though we smiled and laughed, our emotions were drained and really deep inside our hearts began again to fill with sadness. We began to wonder, "Will she get through this? Will she ever grow through the need for all of the care and medical attention that is presently required?"

We were unable to block out the awareness of the tragedy we saw in Hilary. Our only joy was in knowing that a group of gentle and thoughtful people surrounded Hilary, a group of young nurses who were really kindhearted with her, who were willing to do for her whatever she needed.

Perhaps during those first days in General Hospital if someone had done a better job, if someone had been more alert, Hilary would not have acquired the infection that became compounded over the course of a year.

Again, the shunt was working properly. Four days after the party Hilary was released from the hospital.

The winter had been cold. Snow had been accumulating throughout December. I was able to manage the first few snowfalls with a small lawn and garden tractor equipped with a plow but later we had to rely upon a friend with a four-wheel drive truck. After the most immediate snowfall, he worked about two hours and did manage to clear a single lane from the road to the garage. It had been a struggle.

In the meantime, we had obtained electrical components for the furnace should something fail while Hilary was home. Also, we purchased a portable heater and an electric generator if we should lose power. This did happen once the previous year. We were without power for twelve hours. The indoor temperature dropped to fifty degrees. We felt that we were prepared for whatever could possibly happen.

### Daniel J. Dyman, Ed.D.

On Friday morning, eight days after Hilary had come home, the wind began blowing from the East. That was the beginning of a storm that would last through the weekend. As the wind shifted around to the West, drifting intensified as more snow accumulated. By the time the storm was over, eleven inches of snow had fallen. The driveway was filled to the height of my shoulders. We were snowbound. Even our friend with the four-wheel drive truck would be unable to clear the driveway. Our only option was to call an excavator who lived about two miles away.

I explained our situation. God bless him. Lyell agreed to come over with his small bulldozer. The next afternoon, after the main road had been opened, we heard Lyell in the driveway moving the incredible amount of snow. He piled it along the edge of the driveway in some places to a height above our rooftop. We had access to the road if necessary but we would be in serious trouble if another major snowfall were to occur. Fortunately, through the time of the storm, Hilary was at her best.

Hilary appeared to be doing well, she had gained a few more ounces to tip the scales at just over nine pounds, almost as much as she had ever weighed. Charlene was exercising her regularly to help her build up some muscle strength.

Our next goal was to find another pediatric group. We wanted to get away from Drs. Larry, Barney, and Stanley. We obtained the name of the lead doctor that managed Hilary while she was at Community Hospital. But when Charlene contacted Dr. Job, she would have nothing to do with us unless we agreed to get psychological assistance and sign a waiver to not sue for any alleged malpractice.

A lawsuit would never have been an option for us. That consideration would violate the fabric of our character. That we should have to avail ourselves to psychological counseling was insulting. As we saw it, we were mentally alert and determined. None of our actions were offensive and none should have been interpreted as such. We reacted only to what had happened. Obviously, our responses especially mine were misinterpreted and our reputation had circulated throughout the medical community. Almost from the onset we felt marginalized. Now, we felt ostracized.

Consequently, Charlene reestablished contact with Drs. Larry, Barney, and Stanley. This time we were happy to bring Hilary in for an appointment because she was not sick with a cough or temperature, not vomiting or refusing to eat, and it was not at 4:00 p.m. or later just after office closing. Nonetheless, we were not well received. Through the "grapevine" the doctors must have learned that we were shopping for a new group to take care of Hilary.

Upon entering the examination room, Dr. Stanley said, "We knew you'd be back."

Charlene responded, "We were never away. Hilary had surgery to implant a shunt."

Dr. Stanley replied, "Yes, we followed her progress at Community Hospital."

For me, the reply was a verification of my conviction however tentative before.

But, as surprised as I was to hear that answer, I was more astonished as Charlene replied, "Actually, we are glad to hear that. Perhaps the progression of hydrocephalus was the cause of many of Hilary's difficulties, the refusal to eat and the high level of irritability. The postural drainage prescription certainly did not help matters.

"We are just relieved that she is over that hurdle and that we can be here to visit with you while her health is relatively stable. As you can see, she has gained some weight. On the other hand, nine pounds plus a few ounces at just over a year old is not where she should be."

As amazed as I was with Charlene's comment, by his look, Dr. Stanley was staggered. Typically, Charlene had been timid.

Dr. Stanley, still with a look of astonishment, perhaps tinted with guilt, acknowledged that Charlene was correct in her surmise. Then, he turned and began his examination of Hilary, listening to her lungs and heart as well as checking her reflexes. Her eyes did slowly track his hand movements and her arm and leg movements were relaxed.

Nodding his head, Dr. Stanley smiled and said, "She is doing better."

He refilled the prescription for sedative drops and cheerfully said, "Keep up the good work."

For me, that was a shift in disposition. I thanked him and with a smile having gained some approval, we left for home feeling good about what had taken place.

# 17

The day after our visit with Dr. Stanley, the consulting cardiologist's office called complaining that they had not received remuneration for their billing past due three weeks.

Charlene looked into the matter and discovered that the check intended for the cardiologist was endorsed and processed into the account of his associate neurologist whose payment was not due for two more weeks.

I said, "Charlene, what a deal. A true professional business relationship where one partner takes the other guy's money."

Clearly, it was not an error. The payee was clearly identified. Nonetheless, the incident caused a ruckus and of course, it was our fault. We were charged with failure in diligence, paying on time. Our cautious explanation was inadequate. On the spot out of pocket satisfaction was demanded. We had enough. We decided to find another group of doctors who could take care of Hilary.

We felt that our chance of finding this bonanza of sorts was virtually slim to none. But, we did have Dr. Henry's recommendation.

At the risk of losing a portion of our insurance assistance, we decided to go ahead, at least to see if something would work out.

Our meeting with the new doctor on January 26 was easy. We went over Hilary's history. Dr. Overhill examined her. Her abdomen appeared a little distended as we had begun to notice shortly after she had been released from Community Hospital. Dr. Stanley thought it was indicative of a digestive aberration associated with the syndrome by which Hilary was characterized.

## Daniel J. Dyman, Ed.D.

We were relieved when Dr. Overhill told us that he would support us in caring for Hilary. He did not seem concerned with Hilary's distended abdomen. We felt a sense of freedom. We had a place to go.

At the moment, Hilary appeared to be getting along acceptably well. The next two weeks were relatively uneventful. She would fuss from time to time but we continued our program of exercising her that involved no more that working her legs as if she were riding a bicycle and moving her arms as if she were doing jumping jacks or while gently holding her hands tugging on her arms so as to lift her body. Frequently, she would respond as if she wanted to sit up. Those were moments of excitement for us.

In reflection, a lot was taken for granted as Shellie and Therese were growing and developing. Perspectives change dramatically when you have been granted the care of a special child. Any positive response from Hilary was an occasion for celebration always with cheers of delight. Those moments were reinforcements of our hope.

On Valentine's Day, Hilary's behavior deteriorated. Nothing seemed to satisfy her. The next day she was better but fussed a lot more than she usually did. Charlene set up an appointment with her new pediatrician. We had to wait until February 19. Off and on, Hilary would eat a little. She had stopped making progress.

Hilary's abdomen became more firm and distended. This did appear to puzzle Dr. Overhill. He recommended hospitalization to observe her.

Hilary was hospitalized for six days, at a new place for us, Church Hospital. Other than the distension of her abdomen and a refusal to eat, nothing could be discerned from the blood work that had been ordered. Admittedly, Dr. Overhill was baffled.

## Hilary Ann – A Broken Heart

When we arrived to take Hilary home, at 9:00 a.m. on February 25, Charlene checked her chart and nurse's notes. She was elated. Bringing the chart to me she said, "Look. The four o'clock feeding was four ounces. Eight o'clock, four ounces. Wow! We're on track again."

That was good for Hilary. Over the last several days at home, she consumed only between two and three ounces per feeding.

I thought, "Maybe this was the hallmark of something good, a new doctor, a new hospital. This is wonderful!"

Of course, this moment of optimism was tempered by the recollection of the many occasions when Hilary seemed to take a step forward only to be followed by a step or two backward. The setback was before us.

After Hilary had been dressed to go home, we began gathering up her toys and possessions. Charlene reached into the bedside table were she had stowed Hilary's personal file and records. There she discovered a bottle of formula labeled, "Hilary, 4 a.m., 4 oz."

Charlene exclaimed, "What! Somebody has not been truthful. How is it that the chart shows Hilary had consumed four ounces of formula when the four o'clock bottle is still full."

She called for the charge nurse.

Showing both the charted record and the discovered bottle, Charlene said, "Please explain this."

The charge nurse appeared speechless. After moments of hesitation, she said, "Something isn't right here."

Charlene interjected, "Exactly. Whoever wrote this had not been trustworthy. Are any of her charts accurate? Is there anything about her records here that can be relied upon?"

The charge nurse still perplexed replied, "I don't know."

Distraught and disappointed, we signed the release and left for home.

"How incredible!" Charlene exclaimed as we crossed the parking lot making our way to our van.

I answered, "I agree. And, Dr. Overhill should hear about this as well as the hospital administrator. But, does it matter, really? Anyway, whatever is said, the response will always be some list of excuses but nothing acceptable or valid. And, nothing changes. Again, we have been betrayed. Will it always be this way for Hilary again and again?"

Hilary needed the kind of care she received at Community Hospital. That was the bottom line. We would have to submit to the demands of their primary pediatric group. We would have to agree to the psychological assistance program and sign the waiver enjoining a malpractice lawsuit. Simply, we were out of options. We had no choice.

# 18

We tried to manage Hilary but our very best efforts seemed to fall short. Four days after having been released from Church Hospital, Charlene called the pediatric group serving Community Hospital. Fortunately, only the youngest member of the group was in the office, Dr. Noble. Either he was uninformed regarding Dr. Job's proposal in dealing with us or he did not care about the conditions and concerns. Without hesitation or reservation he agreed to see Hilary the next morning.

He said, "Bring her to the hospital examination room on the first floor at ten o'clock. I'll be waiting."

We arrived in the parking lot several minutes early. We were determined to let nothing interfere with our appointment or upset this potential relationship.

As we approached the side entrance to the emergency room, I slipped on an unnoticed patch of ice on the first step above the sidewalk. As I was falling, I cradled Hilary in my arms. In a split second I visualized falling upon her perhaps injuring her. Luckily, I managed to break my fall landing on my right knee and elbow and rolling onto my side. Hilary's head in my hands had been just inches above the concrete. I let out a sigh as I realized that she was safe. Looking at her all bundled up, I whispered, "Thank God that you are okay."

As I got up I let out a deep breath and said to Charlene, "Maybe this will be a day of blessings after all."

She answered with a smile, "Could be."

Though my trousers and coat had gotten soiled I felt so very relieved. Nothing had happened to Hilary. After a moment to regain my composure, we continued on through the outer doors, made a turn following an arrow above a sign pointing us to go down a long hallway. Eventually we found our way to the waiting area adjoining the examination room as agreed. Charlene signed us in. We took a seat. Then, I handed Hilary over to Charlene.

Only seconds had elapsed before Dr. Noble appeared.

He kindly said, "Come this way, please."

We followed him into a small simple essentially empty room. Charlene placed Hilary on a gurney-style table. We gathered around. Our eyes were shifting from Hilary, to the doctor, and to each other.

Gently unwrapping Hilary's blanket and lifting her nightshirt, Dr. Noble said, "So, what do we have here?"

Charlene took out Hilary's file. Though not referring to it, she began to highlight Hilary's history.

After only a few remarks, Dr. Noble interrupted saying, "I'll look into all of that later. I can obtain a copy of her records."

He examined her carefully. Then, in a few moments, looking up to me, he said, "She will have to be admitted."

I answered, "We're always prepared for that."

Dr. Noble directed us to take Hilary to the Pediatrics ward where we felt she had some friends, the nurses who took care of her after her neurosurgery and various shunt revisions.

Hilary was welcomed with warmhearted smiles tempered with expressions of concern. We stayed with her for a few minutes. It was obvious. We were at the mercy of others and fate itself.

I thought, "What more can we do for you child?"

Then, I said to the head nurse, Ms. Susan, "We'll have to go home to get more things for Hilary. We'll be back later tonight or the first thing tomorrow morning."

Almost together, Charlene and I said, "Good-bye, little Hilary Ann."

Ms. Susan could only empathetically smile. But, with that gesture, she did reach out wishing us well.

Again, we left our child with strangers however trusted. It was never easy to turn, to walk out of the hospital leaving behind a most precious little person. Each time, we felt a deep loss.

As I walked through the hallways, my spirit felt empty. I know that Charlene felt the same as I did. We did not turn to each other nor did we say a word. We just walked.

This time as we drove home, we did not have the overwhelming sense of hope as we had the many times before.

We were uncertain and so remained isolated in our thoughts. Dr. Noble seemed caring, different from the others who treated her mechanically. But, we had been so worn down that his concern did not elevate our spirits as otherwise it might have.

As evening approached, I asked Charlene if we could delay our trip back to the hospital until the next day. We had been with Hilary in the morning. We had seen her that day and we were just short of exhausted. Shellie and Therese needed us as well. We spent that evening with both of them.

Shortly after 11:00 p.m., the telephone began to ring. It was Lisa, one of Hilary's nurses. She said, "Mr. Dyman, Hilary isn't doing too well tonight."

I answered, "We plan on coming in tomorrow, first thing in the morning. We'll be bringing some of her things."

Lisa answered with an exceptionally soft voice, "I just called to let you know."

I thanked her for being concerned and went to bed to rest and sleep. I had not figured it out.

At 2:19 a.m., March 3, the ringing telephone awakened me. I got up to answer it. It was, Dr. Noble.

He said quietly with a hesitant voice, "Mr. Dyman, I'm sorry to tell you this but Hilary died just a short time ago."

I exclaimed in disbelief, "Oh my! How could that have happen? I had no idea. Lisa called earlier to say that Hilary was a little dusky and not doing well but frequently since the last shunt revision that's how she had been."

Both of us were silent.

After a few moments, overcome with sadness, choked up almost unable to speak, I said, "I don't know what to do. I don't know how to deal with this."

Still guarded, Dr. Noble replied, "I'm not sure either."

Decidedly shaken with tears forming in my eyes, I said, "Can I call you back in a few minutes? I need some time."

He answered, "Yes. But, in the meanwhile, may I have someone get back to you who may be able to be helpful and who can answer any questions that you have at this time?"

I said, "Thank you."

After I hung up the telephone, I went to wake Charlene but she was already up.

Half asleep, she mumbled, "And, what's that about?"

Distraught, disheartened, dejected, I said, "Hilary died a short time ago."

As I had become, Charlene became, emotionally overcome in disbelief. Tears immediately filled her eyes.

I continued, "Charlene, I'm overwhelmed. I just don't know what to say or do."

I sat down on the edge of the bed next to her. For what seemed to be several minutes, we remained silent.

Disconnected thoughts were passing through my mind but regaining some composure subdued with acceptance, I said, "I have to call my Dad."

Before I could get to the telephone, it began to ring. It was Lisa calling.

Immediately, she graciously said, "Mr. Dyman, I found out some information for you. Mr. O'Brian will come for Hilary about 7:00 a.m. He will take her to his funeral home only a short distance from the hospital on Main Street."

I interjected, "I have no money for this. What might this cost?"

Lisa answered, "I have no idea, Mr. Dyman."

Nonetheless, as Lisa read to me the telephone number of the funeral home, I copied it thinking, "What next?"

She continued in a thoughtful considerate voice, "And, when you come here later, Hilary's belongings will be at the ward clerk's desk. If I can be of anymore help to you, please call me."

I answered, "Oh, no. No. We'll be okay. Thank you."

Lisa replied, "I'm sorry. And, Mr. Dyman, all of us are sorry for the loss of Hilary and do extend our regrets your wife. Please, as you may need, call on anyone of us in the Pediatrics ward."

I replied, "Thank you for all that you have done for us. We really appreciate your compassionate care over the past several weeks. Thank you. And, please thank Dr. Noble for his concern."

We exchanged "Good-bye."

I updated Charlene. She had taken a seat at the dinner table near the kitchen telephone. Then from there, I called my father.

He answered as anyone might, just having been aroused from sleep in the early morning hours, "Hello."

I said, "Dad, this is Dan. I'm sorry to wake you but I'm calling to tell you that Hilary died about an hour ago."

Obviously stunned by what he heard, he responded, "I'm sorry to hear that." Pausing perhaps to gain his composure, he continued, "As you must, remember that all things happen for a reason though you may never know what it is. At this time, important to me is how can I be of help to you and Charlene?"

I thanked him for his thoughtfulness and gave him an account of the last two days. Then I said, "I will be needing your help in this as well as your advice but first, if it is okay with you and Mom, I want to bury Hilary with Arthur."

Arthur was my parents' second child. As a baby, he died from pneumonia. Antibiotics were not yet developed. Had Arthur lived, he would have been my oldest brother. I still had my sister, the oldest, and an older brother. I was the fourth child.

## Hilary Ann – A Broken Heart

My father answered, "That'll be fine. You'll need to call Fr. Lou and John Thomas. I'll see that everything gets done the way you want it. I'm sorry for you and Charlene. I'm sorry that Hilary was unable to make it. She was a special child. I hope that you understand."

Emotionally drained, tears again filling my eyes, I answered, "Could you get the telephone numbers for me?"

In a few minutes, my father gave me two telephone numbers, one for Fr. Lou and the other for John at Thomas Funeral Home. John was a former schoolmate and family friend.

I said, "Thanks for now and I'll be in touch."

My father replied, "I do know how you feel and even how you may be thinking. Take care of yourself and the girls. Give my regards to Charlene. I'll be here for you. Bye now."

I looked over to Charlene. Still in dismay and shaking my head from side to side, I said, "I didn't realize Hilary was dying. Lisa told me that she was not doing well but "was not doing well" means many things. Why didn't she just tell me that Hilary was dying? We needed to be with her. I am so sorry, so very sorry that I did not get it."

Charlene answered, "I know and I understand. And, Hilary knows. It's okay. Our little Hilary will not have to suffer anymore. She's our little angel. We have to believe that. And, isn't it ironic that she died on this date, March 3rd, exactly one year after I expected her to be born."

Quietly Charlene warmed up some coffee. We shared our silence as well. It was too early in the morning to make any more telephone calls. We waited for the sunrise.

# 19

We got the van ready with sleeping bags and breakfast for the girls. We awakened them, Shellie sufficiently alert for a sleep walk. Charlene managed her. Slumped over my shoulder, I carried Therese.

Arriving at the hospital just after 10:00 a.m., we picked up the few things that belonged to Hilary and thanked each of the nurses for their thoughtfulness and generosity. They made a difference for us. They were truly trustworthy. Each offered their consolation, some with tears of their own. We thanked Ms. Susan for her kindness and support.

I remarked. "You have managed to gather a wonderful group of nurses. This is the only hospital where we felt that Hilary received the care that she needed. You and your nursing staff need to know that. Truly, your concern for others and your dedication to the work of your profession make a difference."

Ms. Susan responded, "We are pleased with your comments of appreciation. I will share them with each person here, nurses and staff members as well."

Along with an address, she gave us the directions to get to the funeral home. We said good-bye.

As we were leaving, we were blessed with the unexpected meeting of three of the doctors that had been involved in the care of Hilary one an on-call physician we had met just once, Dr. Stanley, and Dr. David. They were in a conversation in the hallway outside of the Pediatrics ward.

I stopped. They appeared surprised.

I said, "I'm sure that you know Hilary died early this morning."

Each nodded as if to say yes.

I continued, "I feel fortunate to have met you here. Though some times were strained, I do want you to know that I am grateful for what each of you had tried to do for Hilary. Please share my appreciation with your colleagues."

While I was speaking, all kept their heads bowed, looking down. When I had concluded, Dr. David made eye contact with me. Shaking his head expressing a kind of confoundedness, he remarked, "You know, her heart just gave out."

I replied, "Thank you for trying. Certainly, you did give your very best to her. I am most pleased with your effort."

Both Dr. Stanley and his associate remained in their state of detachment. Neither said a word. Perhaps they felt that I was intruding upon their privacy or maybe they did not know what to think or say in response. Thanking them again, I turned away to leave the hospital with Charlene, Shellie and Therese walking hand in hand.

The funeral home was only a mile from the hospital and in the direction of our home. We met briefly with Mr. O'Brian. We explained our needs to which he without hesitation agreed. We would be able to pick up Hilary the next morning and transport her in our van to Thomas Funeral Home for a service before her burial. We left a pink outfit and booties.

Our lives had become dramatically altered. In an instant we had to shift from a dedicated concern for Hilary to the planning of her funeral. Suddenly, we went from a routine of uncertainty and hope to a state of acceptance and finality.

Together, we spent a quiet afternoon and evening. We were physically and emotionally fatigued.

Shellie and Therese must have perceived the somberness in us. Both played quietly. Perhaps Shellie comprehended the loss of Hilary. Certainly, Therese could not grasp the concept. They had to have been weary from another long day of riding in the back of our van. Both went to bed early.

Charlene and I managed to layout the clothes for the girls as well as those that we would wear. Only a few words were spoken. Nothing had to be said. All of the communication that was needed had been in the silence that we kept.

The next morning, earlier than was necessary, still overwhelmed by the events of the last two of days, I was up at just minutes after five o'clock. As I got the van ready, again loading up the breakfast and snacks for Shellie and Therese as well as the games that would occupy them thoughts about Hilary raced through my mind.

I mumbled to myself, "Yes, her heart did give out as Dr. David had said. Surely, it was broken. And, if Hilary had the awareness, she would have felt a broken heart as we had experienced many times before during her short life."

That was an oversimplification. If the doctors had been thoughtful about Hilary, they might have recognized that for the last several weeks, from the time she was released from Community Hospital, she had been in a progressive state of heart failure. Hilary had been accumulating fluid in her abdomen, fluid she could not circulate nor discharge because the blood pressure from her failing heart had become inadequate.

The pediatricians could not see it, not even the cardiologist probably because Hilary was classified in a syndrome box. Always it appeared that placing her into a category was the general preoccupation, the overriding concern. The diagnosis seemed to be more important than Hilary. Consequently, along the way, the many doctors might have realized a lot more than they did. Eventually, I would link the oversight to the hand that destiny had to play.

Hilary's entire life was a tragedy founded upon a series of errors and oversights and albeit even an occasional touch of neglect and selfishness. Except for a few, everyone everywhere likely did their best but somehow failed her. And, among those that could have done more, a few perhaps with a touch of malevolence may have deliberately overlooked this child with special needs. But, as I discovered, only an occasional person is uniquely prepared to understand and care for children in this select group. Apart from Dr. Edwards and perhaps Dr. Noah as well as Dr. Noble only the nurses at Community Hospital truly demonstrated empathy for Hilary and shared with her a portion of their compassion. I would often wonder, "Why?"

As we drove, our conversation became a litany of events. We recalled some of the rare joyful moments sprinkled in with every slight and every hurtful incident. Our devastating frustration was contained only by the realization that no one could ever again hurt Hilary with some kind of inappropriately determined treatment. But, then no one could care for her or fuss over her needs. A vacancy that could never be filled now existed for us.

We arrived just after 9:00 a.m. Mr. O'Brian greeted us in the foyer of the funeral home and asked us to be seated. We waited for maybe five minutes before he returned. He led us to the viewing parlor.

At the end of the dimly lighted somber room we saw Hilary. She was dressed in her pink outfit lying in a pink casket, a burning candle placed at either end. The candles appeared to glow softly surrendering their flickering light while at the same time creating solemn ethereal images all around. A bouquet of flowers had been set to the back of the casket over the open lid in the center of which was placed a small crucifix. The flowers were from the pediatric nurses at Community Hospital.

Shellie and Therese slowly approached the casket apparently not knowing what to make of what they were seeing. Shellie was tall enough but Therese had to stand on her toes to see Hilary. Shellie slipped a folded paper into the casket along side Hilary.

It read,
    God, I'm sorta happy that Hilary died.
    But I liked Hilary a lot.
    I liked when I held her.
    I really didn't want her to die.
    I guess that's the way it is.
        Love, Shellie Dyman

On the bottom, Shellie had drawn a head stone with a cross and the name, Hilary.

After Charlene and I had read the words seeing them for the first time, we replaced Shellie's note as she had put it next to Hilary. In addition, we tucked a small pink teddy bear next to Hilary inside of her left arm. We stepped back and stood silent absorbing the preciousness of the scene that was before us. It would forever stay fixed in our memory. Words could not express the feelings we had. The tears in our eyes spoke our thoughts, the loss we realized with the sense of peace that somehow prevailed. Hilary was at rest.

The gentle closing of a door behind us shifted our attention. As we turned, we saw that it was Mr. O'Brian.

I walked to him. I said, "Thank you for all that you have done for us. What do we owe you for these services?"

Mr. O'Brian answered, "There are no charges."

I replied, "Surely, there must be some cost to you for your time, your effort here, and at least for the casket."

Mr. O'Brian responded, "Simply, there are no charges. We are grateful that we could be of assistance to you and your family."

With a smile communicating my most sincere appreciation, I said, "Thank you for your kindness. It does mean a lot to Charlene and to me."

Mr. O'Brian smiled in return and shook my hand. He said, "Here are the papers that you will need to transport Hilary. And, be careful on the road. You have to be stressed over the loss of your daughter. So, do not hurry along and again, please be careful as you drive."

I answered saying, "Thank you. Thank you very much."

Mr. O'Brian took me by the arm. We were led to the foyer. Mr. O'Brian said, "I'll be just a few minutes."

When he returned, Hilary was closed in her casket on a small bier. With all of us walking along side the casket, Mr. O'Brian proceeded to our van and placed the casket in the same space where Hilary's car bed used to be between the two bucket-type front seats. Then he went to get the bouquet of flowers. These he placed out of the way behind the driver's seat but close to Hilary's casket.

I said, "Thank you, Mr. O'Brian. "Thank you so much for everything and most of all for your consideration and kindness."

With an honest expression of concern, Mr. O'Brian said, "You're welcome. Again, drive carefully."

We got into the van and began our two and one half hour drive to Thomas Funeral Home where we would meet family and friends.

# 20

We arrived at Thomas Funeral Home just after noon. The day was overcast. The air was filled with a cool mist.

After we got out of the van, I lifted Hilary's casket from between the front seats.

Very softly I said, "Hilary, before we used to drive with you in panic. Today, it was different. You were in peace in a different place now as God's little angel. Remember us, Hilary. We tried. I'm truly sorry if ever I had failed you."

The casket with Hilary was not heavy. Of course, in life, she never had weighed very much.

Charlene carrying the flowers, the girls walking along, led the way. At the entrance, Shellie held open the door. As soon as I had entered, John Thomas met me and directed me to a small parlor. I placed the casket on a small bier that was surrounded on three sides by wreaths and bouquets of flowers sent by members of our family as well as friends even by students in my classes and colleagues in my department.

It was an emotional moment. Tears came to my eyes but I had to maintain my composure. I could not cause a scene. Others in the gathering appeared to be on the brink of an emotional break down.

Cards of sympathy were given to Charlene and to me, some contained money to help defray expenses. In total, the various gifts that we received in Hilary's memory covered all of the funeral expenses except for twenty dollars, the cost of digging her grave. Ironically, while we were unable to acquire insurance for such expenses, we were the benefactors of the generosity of family, friends, and even strangers.

## Hilary Ann – A Broken Heart

My brother came to me and said, "I'm sorry but you have to feel relieved that this burden has been lifted from your shoulders."

I knew that my brother's remark had been well intended. The last fourteen months with Hilary were not easy. Just the same, it stung a bit and I felt offended by it.

I responded, "Yes, but Hilary was my daughter. She could never be a burden."

After my response, I had hoped that he understood. Indeed we had many restless nights and anxious moments. We faced times of frustration. But, Hilary was so dear to Charlene and to me, I am absolutely sure that any burden she could ever be would have been veiled just by her presence.

I thought, "No matter how difficult, Hilary was our child. During her short life, we struggled more than perhaps we experienced joy and happiness. Maybe those gifts were present but we were unable to recognize either of them. We would never know her as she might be but she had been and will always be a special treasure given to us. In her need, we had become bonded to her. I hoped that Charlene and I had been for her all that we needed to be. I hoped that she would see us as having given to her all that we could possibly give."

Fr. Lou led a brief funeral service of prayers and offered a homily. He spoke about the presence of God in our lives, that in ways unknown to us He is with us. It is our response to our situation that determines the extent of our Faith and the measure of our trust.

At the conclusion of the service, I carried Hilary back to our van and placed her for the last time between the two front seats.

A formal funeral procession had not been planned. We gathered at the cemetery at the place that had been set a side for Hilary. One by one, the cars of people arrived. When everyone gathered around the burial site, I carried Hilary from the van and placed her casket on the ground next to the place where she would be buried. We prayed for those who had gathered.

The scene was austere, the air brisk, cold and damp. The trees without their leaves stood as eerie bending and swaying silhouettes against the backdrop of a swiftly moving gray sky. The people with heads bowed perhaps in bewilderment perhaps in contemplation of what they in a short time had witnessed, sprinkled flower petals on Hilary's casket. Then, each began to step away going to their cars.

I felt a little tug on my topcoat. It was Therese. I looked down to her.

She said, "Pick up Hilary, Daddy. Pick up Hilary."

Charlene gently took Therese by the hand and bending down to her softly said, "Hilary will be okay. It's okay, Therese. We need to go home where we can remember her."

Charlene with Therese in hand pulling her along began to slowly walk toward the van. Therese looking back over her shoulder toddling over the grass almost stumbling as only a two year old might do surely had been unable to understand that Hilary would not be coming home.

I stayed behind. I wanted to be present until Hilary had been placed into her grave and dirt covered her casket. I wanted to be with her until the last moment.

I needed to say to her, "I'm sorry for not being with you when you died, when you may have needed me more than at any other time, when I needed you most of all. Nothing would have changed but I wanted to be there for you. Had I only known, I would have been with you."

## Hilary Ann – A Broken Heart

The young man who had dug Hilary's grave approached from several yards away. When he came close, I could see that he was afflicted with Down's syndrome. It was fitting that he should be here for Hilary. He was gentle, kind, and considerate.

Without a spoken word, by someone I could not have expected, I had been consoled. He seemed to me to be a messenger of that peacefulness. Surely, the least among us shall be first. The merits of the challenged, afflicted, and deprived are beyond comprehension. I would be forever grateful that he had stood near me.

On his knees, as if in prayer, he carefully picked up the casket, reached over the grave, and gently lowered Hilary into the earth. I took his shovel and slowly sprinkled dirt over the top of her casket that had been covered by the delicate blanket of flower petals left by those who only moments ago said farewell.

He interrupted me saying, "I will finish this for you."

With tears streaming down my face, I handed over the shovel saying with a choked up voice that almost could not make a sound, "Thank you. She's special."

I turned and left Hilary where she is. I believed as I would always believe, "You are safe, Hilary. Each day you will be in our life in some way and someday we will meet again to truly know each other."

We drove home, emptied of every emotion. Again, our conversation focused on days and events in Hilary's short life, events that brought happiness and those that brought disappointment, anxiety, frustration, and sadness.

We ordered a stone to mark Hilary's grave. Across the top would be etched, Hilary Ann Dyman. Below and in the center a plain cross, to the left her birth date and on the right the date of her death. The stone would be fashioned after the sketch Shellie had added at the bottom of her letter sent with Hilary to God.

However, when we returned to the gravesite exactly one month after Hilary had died, we found that the stone had been poorly placed, tilted and out of alignment. It had to be repositioned. And, as a symbol of our remembrance, we planted bulbs of pretty little pink flowers to cover her resting place. During the springtime, only a few had sprouted and by the end of summer, all had died.

Charlene and I concluded, "That seemed fitting. As in life so be it after death."

# 21

On March 14, eleven days after Hilary had died we received the following letter from Community Hospital:

> Dear Mr. & Mrs. Dyman:
>
> Although you may not know us well, we at Community Hospital participated in the care of someone close to you. We extend to you our deepest sympathy at the loss of your daughter.
>
> Each patient is very special to us, deserving personal care and comfort. Though we could not prevent your grief, we want you to know that we tried to do so to the best of our abilities. We hope that our attention was able to make the passing more peaceful and free from strife.
>
> Like you, we share in the disappointment that even the most advanced medical knowledge cannot always provide a cure. We can only offer you our most sincere condolences, and a thought from British writer Samuel Butler:
>
> "To die completely, a person must not only forget but be forgotten, and he who is not forgotten is not dead."
>
> May God watch over you and those you love, now and throughout the year.
>
> Sincerely,
>
> Noel Goode
> President

The letter awoke the memories we had of Hilary and of the care that she inspired during her last days. She had been for us a dear child never to be forgotten. The letter renewed all of our realizations. But, on July 5, from the Community

Daniel J. Dyman, Ed.D.

Hospital Business Office, we received an invoice with a cover letter. The invoice and letter were as follows:

| Patient Name | Account No. | Am't |
|---|---|---|
| Hilary Dyman | 73803047 | $ 229.80 |

Dear Mr. Dyman:

The above account is long overdue.

Please contact us immediately to arrange a satisfactory payment agreement on your account.

If we do not hear from you within fifteen (15) days from the date of this letter, we will have no alternative but to consider proceeding with the legal remedies available to us. Should we recover a Judgment against you, we would consider execution by the attachment of your property, and the garnishment of your bank accounts and earnings.

Yours very truly,

COMMUNITY HOSPITAL
By: Mr. Mand

The invoice had been stamped "This account has been assigned for collection. Pay in full at once. We will withhold action for seven (7) days."

I was distraught when I read the letter and looked over the details of the invoice.

As I showed the account document and letter of notification to Charlene, I said, "Look! This is crazy. For a few hundred dollars they want to attach my paycheck or house which ever comes first. It's awful. How much have we already paid them?"

Charlene interrupted, "We don't owe anything. I have a statement that indicates that all is paid in full."

I responded, "Then this is some kind of a mistake. I'll call this guy, Mand, and we'll get this straightened out right now."

I picked up the telephone and dialed the number at the top in the letterhead.

After two rings, the voice at the other end answered, "Community Hospital Business Office."

I replied, "Hi, my name is Daniel Dyman. I just received a letter and statement from your office indicating that you are planning action against me for not having paid $229.80 on account number 73803047. According to my wife, our records show that our account with you is closed, marked paid in full."

The person to whom I was speaking replied, "Oh. I can't do anything about that. The person you need to speak with is Mr. Mand."

I said, "Well, may I speak with him."

The person answered, "He is not available right now."

I responded, "Obviously, I need to speak with him. When will he be available?"

The person replied, "I don't know that. You can try later."

As I said, "Thank you," I heard the telephone being hung up.

Surprised by the lack of politeness, I said to Charlene, "The person that I need to speak with isn't available. I have to try later. I can't believe this."

Charlene replied, "It shouldn't be a problem. We'll work it out."

I called Mr. Mand two more times that morning, once just before noon. Each time, I spoke with the same person who gave me the same response, "He is not available. Call later."

I called three more times in the afternoon and was given the same response as if it were a recorded message. Now, 4:30 p.m., I called again. Again, I received the same answer. But, by this time, I had become upset. The letter was specific, "Please contact us immediately."

I had tried throughout the day. I called five minutes later. This time a different person answered the telephone.

I politely said, "I need to speak with Mr. Mand.

The person responded, "He's somewhere. He's been busy all day with movers changing the layout of the office."

On hearing that he was rearranging his office, I became openly angry. I said, "Please, will you let him know that I have been calling him all day about an urgent matter. I need to speak with him."

The person answered, "I'll give him the message. Thank you."

However, before she could hang up the telephone, I added, "Now, understand. He needs to call me. For me, this is a matter of great urgency."

I hung up the telephone, turned to Charlene, and said, "I just cannot accept what is happening. I get this awful letter. I call repeatedly all throughout the day to learn that Mr. Mand is not available to me because he is arranging his office furniture."

I was burning with fury but I waited watching as minutes ticked off the clock.

At 4:53 p.m., I picked up the telephone and re-dialed Mr. Mand's office number.

The first person I had spoken to who throughout the day said, "Mr. Mand is not available," answered my call.

Before she could complete the phrase "Community Hospital Business Office," I broke in saying, "All day I tried to speak with Mr. Mand. He had been unavailable to me. All day I stressed over his letter threatening the possible attachment of my house. Then I discovered that he had been available in his office throughout the day absorbed in rearranging his furnishings and fixtures. Well, you tell Mr. Mand that tomorrow he will find a full-page ad in the local newspaper. On the top, will appear the letter from Mr. Goode expressing condolences over the death of my daughter. Immediately below that will appear the letter and account notice I received from Mr. Mand. And, below that will appear a paid in full statement with a note about your rudeness and his obliviousness over a matter of concern. I promise you. This will happen."

Without any closing remark, I hung up the telephone.

Within seconds, before I had been able to walk from my home office into the kitchen, the telephone began to ring.

Upon picking up the telephone, I said, "Hello."

I heard, "Mr. Dyman, this is Mr. Mand at Community Hospital. I am sorry for any inconvenience that you experienced. I had been rearranging the office and lost track of the important calls that should have been made."

Calmly and quietly, I responded, "Thank you for returning my call. About this letter and statement I received from your office, our records show that this account is closed, paid in full. I need for you to verify that. Can you do that by the end of business tomorrow?"

He replied, "Yes, thank you for your understanding."

The next day we received the following letter:

> Dear Friends:
>
> There is a premise upon which my life is built and upon which I function: "God is too loving to be unkind and too wise to make a mistake." May there be comfort and peace for you from that truth in the loss of Hilary.
>
> The apology offered on the telephone is only being strengthened in this letter. The error in action taken by Community Hospital cries out too loudly and I am sorry for any complications caused for you.
>
> The account sent to the Collection Service Bureau has been cancelled and removed. Any balance on Hilary's last inpatient account will be paid by your insurance.
>
> Thank you for your understanding, patience and forgiveness. Community Hospital continues to be a haven for those needing quality care with tender loving care added.
>
> Sincerely<br>Everett Mand<br>Financial Assistance Manager

Finally, it was over. The proverbial last "t" had been crossed and the last "i" had been dotted.

# EPILOGUE

After Hilary's funeral, when I had returned to teaching on Monday, March 7, an envelope was handed to me. The following was written on the single sheet of paper it contained:

### God's Lent Child – God's Loan

I'll lend you for a little time
A child of mine God said
For you to love the while she lives
And mourn for when she's dead.

It may be six or seven years
Or forty-two or three
But will you, till I call her back
Take care of her for me?

She'll bring her charms to gladden you
And should her stay be brief
You'll have her lovely memories
As a solace for your grief.

I cannot promise she will stay
Since all from earth return
But there are lessons taught down there
I want this child to learn.

I've looked this whole world over
In my search for teachers true
And from the throngs that crowd life's lanes
I have chosen you.

Now will you give her all your love
Nor think the labor vain
Nor hate me when I come to take
This lent child back again?

## Daniel J. Dyman, Ed.D.

> I fancied that I heard them say
> "Dear Lord," Thy will be done
> For all the joys Thy child will bring
> The risk of grief we'll run.
>
> We will shelter her with tenderness
> We'll love her while we may
> And for the happiness we've known
> Forever grateful stay.
>
> But should the angels call for her
> Much sooner than we've planned
> We'll brave the bitter grief that comes
> And try to understand.
>
> Anon

During the second week of July, as the year before, I attended a six-day international conference titled Health Care, Ethics, and Human Values.

The topics included: The Philosophy and Theology of Medicine; Medicine in the History and the Idea of Man; Theories of Justice and their Applicability to Health-Care Delivery; Mental Health of Western Societies; and Who Speaks for the Helpless Child.

The format of the conference enabled individuals like myself to meet and converse with the presenters during breakfast, lunch, and evening buffets.

I enjoyed the opportunities. I was interested in theology, philosophy, and ethics. My undergraduate degree included a minor in philosophy. And, our society was on the frontier in organ transplants, genetic and fetal research, and realizations in coping with death and dying as well as mental illness.

# Hilary Ann – A Broken Heart

Think tanks were being developed for the advancement of wisdom needed for good decision-making. Articles and books had been coming from everywhere. Included among the many published books of interest to me were: *The Medical Nemesis*; *Science, Ethics and Medicine*; *Bioethics and Human Rights*; and *Come, Let Us Play God*.

During one of the evening buffets, I shared my dinner with a notable in psychiatry. Others who were seated at the table were a law school dean, a clergyman, and another interested person not unlike myself.

As the conversation shifted from topic to topic, I offered some firsthand experience about Hilary's treatment, primarily those segments that I perceived as a disregard for her well-being and the continuous effort to exclude Charlene and me from the essential participatory processes.

I commented that once I could not help but listen to a telephone conversation that intensified my determination to never yield on the issues of my responsibility as a parent. Through a partially open door, I overheard one doctor say to another, "Well, we'll just have to provide the information in such a way so that they (referring to Charlene and me) will not have a choice."

Suddenly, the psychiatrist who was seated to my right firmly grabbed my arm just above the wrist. I was immobilized with the force that he exerted coupled with trepidation thinking that I had said something out of line.

As I turned to him, with indisputable intensity, he looked straight into my eyes and said, "Sue the bastards for five million dollars. Not for what they did to your daughter but for the mental cruelty they imposed upon you and your wife. We need a lawsuit like that in our country."

The people around the table were speechless, appearing as stunned as I was. The lawyer who when I had been relating events seemed to roll his eyes saying with his body language, "Oh, please," suddenly appeared taken aback.

The psychiatrist released his grip on my arm. Still in eye contact with me, he added, "I'm serious. We need a lawsuit like this."

Regaining my composure, clearing my throat, I responded, "I'm not sure that I could deal with it."

After a few moments of silence, we went on with our dinner. Nothing related to any of the conference issues was mentioned again that evening around the table.

Charlene and I never did file the recommended lawsuit.

First, it was not in our make up contrary perhaps to the suspicions of some of Hilary's doctors although some may have earned the right to be sued.

Second, we felt that living the events in Hilary's life were enough and neither of us had the spirit to deal with all of the "I say - You say" haggling that might come about and the stress that might result.

Third, if we were to win a judgment or if we were able to negotiate a settlement, the money would likely come from a third party payer and neither Charlene nor I were certain that the outcome would lead to any alteration in the behaviors of those who perhaps poorly or inadvertently cared for Hilary. It was our assumption that those individuals would not recognize a need for reflection or for change. They might even become more indifferent toward others like Hilary and conceivably would have a foundation upon which to justify their callousness.

Fourth, we agreed that the amount of money, whatever the amount, would be no use. We would rather live the remainder of our lives without than indulge ourselves with the equivalent of what we saw to be "thirty pieces of silver."

## Hilary Ann – A Broken Heart

The events that followed the birth of Hilary could never have been anticipated. But, with the additive impact of each complication, we grew to accept Hilary as she was. We did not expect any miracles nor did we expect a cure. We did not expect anyone to play the role of God. We did expect that those who chose a career in the medical profession would measure up to the bottom line of general expectations; that they would as with anyone else value her and care about her, a challenged child; that they would be for her what she needed; that they would be tolerant and kind, considerate and honest, as well as understanding and truthful. We expected that their work performance would at least measure up to what they claimed in payment. We expected nothing more than what seemed reasonable and asked for nothing more than what appeared to be due.

Most of the time that Hilary was hospitalized, she was in a special care unit. The bills were substantial by any standard. She was to have received one-on-one care. But presumably, Hilary may have received no more than what occurs in the wild when a less-than-self-sufficient variant is born. It is quickly destroyed either by its own kind or by awaiting predators. That may seem harsh but along the way we came to believe that often Hilary had been neglected and at times may have been mistreated at least through a lack of concern. We felt that some even looked upon her with disdain. Why? Were not all pledged to care giving?

In all, Hilary was hospitalized one hundred and ninety-one days, just under forty-six per cent of her life. She was treated in five different hospitals, had been in some way touched by at least eighty-five doctors, and had been tended to by countless nurses. Of these only one hospital truly had a caring staff and while a few doctors seemed to have sincerely tried and gave their best effort, only one truly understood. Was it because his child died during heart surgery?

We experienced the failures and consequences of human flaws and defects among the professionals that were

## Daniel J. Dyman, Ed.D.

encountered. No doubt, some did not comprehend frailty; some led by curiosity focused on the science of treatment; and some perhaps out of conditioning were confined in the boundaries of detachment. Surely, while no one may have acted intending harm, the blend of qualities and personalities, the mix of pluses and minuses, indeed led to Hilary's demise.

After considerable reflection upon the events in Hilary's life and several unrelated personal experiences, arguably all would be better for it if the word patient no longer were used in reference to those seeking assistance from medical professionals of every kind and at every level. Individuals should be known by their names rather than by a general category into which they might be assigned.

Its use, media influenced intentionally or inadvertently, defines the authoritative superiority of a group, a select set, who by degree no doubt honorably earned and credentialed by mandate can exclusively dominate and specify the submissive role of all others, a disadvantaged and dependent category set in the framework of discipline limited knowledge and access restrictions. In that context, the potential for collaborative and interactive accommodation necessary for positive caring relationships is countermanded.

Likely, this needs to be accomplished in a framework of humility that is not recognized through a display of stooped shoulders and downtrodden appearance. Rather, humility is the recognition of true personal worth without association to arrogance or conceit.

Those privileged health care providers at all levels have within their grasp the discretion to provide or withhold treatments and services and the capacity to seize complete responsibility for what is clearly the rightful domain of every individual, their physical and even mental well-being.

Those in the medical business are not expected to be healers divinely or otherwise empowered to cure every affliction or malady rather they are expected to be helpful in alleviating the impact of mishap, infection, or shortfall of nature. They are attested attendants along the way of the life journey we share. They need to mediate productive associations whereby all avenues of recourse are made known without bias thus enabling freely exercised choice. Never to be skewed according to personal preference, all options need to be openly explored, evaluated, and explained so that individuals may knowingly select for themselves.

Errors may occur and misfortune may be forthcoming but the range of power is clearly hand in hand linked to responsibility that is directly proportionate to accountability.

What is needed is a fundamental conferment of reverence the entitlement of each individual not earned but endowed within the essence their being. Accordingly, all are equal and thus all are deserving of a rightful high regard and unconditional heart-centered esteem.

I found when in the sixth grade, now on a tattered piece of paper from then on having been in my billfold, a verse that deserves daily reflection. It follows:

### Kindness

I shall pass this way but once, any good things therefore that I can do or any kindness that I can show to any human being, let me do it now. Let me not defer it or neglect it, for I shall not pass along this way again.

Anon

A single day has not gone by without some thought of Hilary. How would she look? What would interest her? How would she be occupied? Had she lived, how would we share each of the remaining days? Forever, we will never know.

ISBN 1425136125